THE pH MIRACLE
FOR DIABETES

THE pH MIRACLE FOR DIABETES

The Revolutionary Diet Plan for Type 1 and Type 2 Diabetics

Robert O. Young, Ph.D., and Shelley Redford Young

Foreword by Chi C. Mao, M.D., Ph.D.

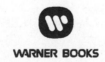

WARNER BOOKS

NEW YORK   BOSTON

Warner Books

Time Warner Book Group
1271 Avenue of the Americas, New York, NY 10020
Visit our Web site at www.twbookmark.com.

Printed in the United States of America

First Printing: July 2004
10 9 8 7 6 5 4 3 2 1

Library of Congress Cataloging-in-Publication Data

Young, Robert O.
    The pH miracle for diabetes : the revolutionary diet plan for Type 1 and Type 2 diabetics / Robert O. Young and Shelley Redford Young.
        p. cm.
    Includes index.
    ISBN 0-446-53266-5
    1. Diabetes—Diet therapy.   2. Hydrogen-ion concentration.   3. Acid-base imbalances—Complications.   I. Young, Shelley Redford.   II. Title.
    RC662.Y68 2004
    616.4'620654—dc22

                                                        2004001644

Book design by Giorgetta Bell McRee

Dedication

To my mother, Lois Young, who passed away this last year. My mother was a great example of patience, persistence, and long suffering and taught me by her words and by her deeds the importance and value of hard work, having faith and trust in our fellow man and, most important, having an abiding faith, trust, and love in Our Heavenly Father.

To my wife, Shelley, who has always been my inspiration to be excellent in all things, just as she is excellent. And to my wonderful and beautiful children: Adam, Ashley, Andrew, and Alex. And to our son-in-law, Mathew, and our healthy pH Miracle grandson, CharLee.

I truly trust and believe in the words of the Prophet David O. Mckay, "No success in life can compensate for a failure in the home." I can truly say that I am a blessed man and a successful man because I have the most incredible family in the world! Each member of our family has been a blessing in my life. Each member of our family is incredibly talented and gifted. And each member of our family is a beacon of light and truth to their center of influence.

To Antoine Bechamp. If his profound voice and science had not been silenced, much of humankind may have been spared the worst aspects of the infectious and degenerative diseases—including diabetes Type 1 and 2—of the twentieth century.

To our future—the children of the world who are at the forefront of an ever-changing and challenging world. Diabetes is now the fastest growing illness in the children of the world. We all need to be unified in stopping and slowing down this epidemic. It is my hope and prayer that the message of *The pH Miracle for Diabetes* will be received by mothers, fathers, teachers, and clergy who will then teach the children this new way of living, eating, and thinking and save our children from unnecessary pain and suffering.

And finally to the American Indians who are the descendants of Mannasseh, the brother of Ephraim whose father was Joseph of old who was sold into Egypt. These are the original heirs of this great American continent and part of the lost tribes of Israel. To them I extend my hand, my heart, and my help to those who are suffering the most from diabetes.

Acknowledgments

No good act performed in the world ever dies. No atom of matter can ever be destroyed. No force, once started, ever ends; it merely passes through a multiplicity of ever-changing phases. This is what I call the doctrine of pleomorphism, or the law of change.

Every good deed done to others is a great force that starts an unending pulsation through time and all eternity. We may not know it, we may never hear a word of gratitude or of recognition in our lifetime, but it will all come back to us in some form as naturally, as perfectly, as inevitably, as an echo answers to sound. Perhaps not as we expect it, how we expect it, nor where; but sometime, somehow, somewhere, it comes back, as the dove that Noah sent from the Ark returned with its green leaf of revelation.

I perceive of gratitude in its largest, most beautiful sense, that if I receive any kindness I am a debtor, not merely to one man or woman but to the whole world. As I am each day indebted to thousands for the comforts, joys, successes, consolations, peace, love, and blessings of life, I realize that it is only by kindness to all that I can begin to repay the debt to one and begin making gratitude the atmosphere of all my living, and a constant companion of expression in outward acts of kindness rather than in mere thoughts.

The pH Miracle for Diabetes is a beginning work of not just mere thoughts or theories but an outward expression of my gratitude for thousands of folks who helped me along my journey toward understanding diabetes, working toward a cure, and then expressing my work in words that could hopefully be understood by everyone.

My gratitude and thanks begin with Dr. William Crook, who impressed and enlightened me with his work on yeast infections and their connection to hyper- and hypoglycemia and diabetes, as expressed in his book *The Yeast Connection*. Inspired by Dr. Crook's work, as early as 1988, I suggested that diabetes was a yeast infection of the pancreas associated with brewer's yeast (*Saccharomyces cerevisiae*) found in the baked goods that many of us eat every day.

Dr. Crook introduced me to another great doctor and researcher, Dr. Orian Truss, and his book *The Missing Diagnosis,* who also suggested that high titers of yeast are associated with hypo- and hyperglycemia, and diabetes. Here now were two witnesses declaring a possible cause for diabetes. I knew if I could understand the cause of diabetes then I could possibly find a cure. This was now my dream, inspired by these two great medical doctors willing to take a risk to think and act outside the orthodox medical box.

In 1994, two incredible events happened. First, I was introduced to the work of Dr. A. V. Constantini and his book *The Fungal/ Mycotoxin Etiology of Human Disease.* Dr. Constantini suggested that the mycotoxin alloxan, which is derived from uric acid, which is then generally derived from animal proteins, is the poison or acid that destroys the insulin-producing beta cells, setting the stage for diabetes. Dr. Constantini was associating the waste product, or acid, from yeast to the cause of beta cell breakdown. I was so thankful at the time for this research because it prepared me to understand what I was about to witness in a twenty-one-year-old Type 1 diabetic— the biological transmutation of a red blood cell to a bacterial cell, like anthraxus bacillus.

As discussed in chapter 1, the biological transmutation of red blood cells I witnessed in this young diabetic woman was a monumental gift that helped me understand the nature of matter, the universal law of change, and the contextual cause of diabetes for which I will be eternally grateful.

From these two revealing events I established the foundation of my theory for diabetes. That is, diabetes is not a disease of the insulin-producing beta cells or pancreas incapable of producing or regulating insulin and glucose but a pH imbalance—overacidity—in the fluids that surround the insulin-producing beta cells or alpha cells that causes them or the pancreas to dysfunction or malfunction.

I will always be grateful to my mentor and hero, Dr. Antoine Bechamp, who has changed my life forever and inspired me with his works *The Blood and Its Third Anatomical Element* and *Les Micro-zymas,* where he drew with his own hand, over one hundred years ago, the biological transmutation of the human cell. I began to cry when I saw his drawings of biological transmutation for the first time, because I knew now I was not alone in my theories and observations.

I am honored to have a foreword by a man of the stature of Chi C. Mao, M.D., Ph.D., and scientist, previously at the National Institutes of Health. Dr. Mao lives and works in Houston, Texas, the same place where I made my first discoveries of pleomorphism in the spring of 1994 and documented its reality. I believe his foreword is no coincidence, but destiny. Dr. Mao has the insight and the courage to stand up for the truth in a world that is full of people who would rather side with what is traditional, convenient, and comfortable. Why would anyone want to rock the boat? Because doing so is changing—saving—lives. Thank you, Dr. Mao, for your beautiful and truthful foreword. This book would not be complete without your words.

To the thousands of diabetics worldwide and to the participants of two controlled diabetic studies who were courageous enough to apply the recommended principles of health and fitness contained in this book and make the necessary lifestyle and dietary changes to slow down, reverse, and even cure their diabetes, I am truly thankful. You are all an inspiration of patience, persistence, faith, hope, and dedication, not only to me but to all who will read and understand the research and your stories. It will be through your testimonies of success, your individual experiences in reversing your diabetes, that thousands, if not hundreds of thousands, of other lives will be changed forever, saved from this unnecessary disease.

To our editor Colleen Kapklein, who carefully and thoughtfully took on my scientific work and words on diabetes and helped me express it in a better way, with the hope that all who would read *The pH Miracle of Diabetes* would improve the quality and the quantity of life by applying the principles contained therein.

To our publisher Warner Books, and Diana Baroni, senior editor for Warner Books: my heartfelt thanks and gratitude for having the faith, courage, and vision to publish not just another book on diabetes but a book that will now empower people to prevent and move beyond their symptoms of diabetes.

To our children, Adam, Ashley, Andrew, and especially Alex, our youngest, for their encouragement, support, and sacrifices as their father and mother took time away from their lives to help and serve others. I am grateful to have children who know who they are and how much they are loved.

And finally, but not least, may I express my gratitude and thanks to my eternal companion, in this life and the life to come, for her constant caring, love, and support for me and this work, even at the expense of her own personal interests. An incredible artist, Shelley will put down her paintbrush for a time so she can serve others in need, in this incredible mission of healing. Her contributions to *The pH Miracle for Diabetes,* of how to live and eat, are lifesaving to the diabetic or prediabetic. Without her creative knowledge and common sense there would be no cure for diabetes, considering we all have to eat to live!

Shelley has created many new incredible recipes included in this book that taste good and not only contribute to the health of the diabetic but to anyone who is seeking outstanding health. In addition, there are also many delicious recipes contributed by the participants of the pH Miracle recipe contest held July 2003, which we have gratefully included.

Shelley is the perfect example of thanks-doing, gratitude, sacrifice, selflessness, and love, all attributes of a Christ-like person. What more could a man ask God for? I am and will be eternally grateful to God for creating such a beautiful soul whom I have the gift and privilege to share life with.

In love, gratitude, and thanksgiving,
Dr. Robert O. Young

Contents

Foreword

According to mainstream medicine, diabetes mellitus, either type 1 (which can be controlled by direct insulin injection) or type 2 (which also may be controlled by oral medication to stimulate insulin production) has long been considered incurable. Physicians have been taught as such and patients are informed as such. Despite the fact that the scope of medications for diabetes has been expanding rapidly, the disease has now reached epidemic proportions, sadly more so among our younger generations. Practitioners in this field cannot help but wonder where we have gone wrong and what we should do to better manage this disease.

In his book *The pH Miracle for Diabetes*, Dr. Robert O. Young presents a comprehensive approach to this disease and aims for a complete cure: what modern medicine would claim as an unthinkable goal. Over the years, through Dr. Young's clinical experience, his studies in this field, as well as numerous positive testimonials from his patients and mine, Dr. Young's approach has been proven to be both medically viable and extremely exciting. In this book, Dr. Young has created a working manual for managing ailments associated with diabetes—and he may even offer a path for a cure.

Dr. Young's House of Health is built on a foundation of acid–base balance, or pH balance. Overacidification of our body fluids, due to our diet and modern lifestyles, is the origin of myriad illnesses; therefore, in order to regain our health, it becomes imperative to minimize acidification and restore a critical balance. Indeed, this theory reminds me of ancient Chinese medical philosophy. Thousands of years ago, health care providers in China already knew that the maintenance of a delicate balance between opposite forces in life—yin and yang, hot and cold, fullness and deficiency, albeit in abstract terms—was essential for human health. Different therapeutic measures such as herbal medicine, acupuncture, body manipulation (massage), and qi-gong were used to restore these balances. It would be interesting to ponder if pH balance is actually a modern scientific expression of this ancient medical philosophy.

Vitamins, minerals, antioxidants, and other essential nutrients from food and supplements have been recognized as crucial to the maintenance of health, as well as for slowing the aging process. In this book, a great deal of attention is paid to these substances, particularly in light of their beneficial effects on diabetes. Through scientific research conducted in recent years, aging, which is commonly viewed as an unavoidable natural process, can now be considered a syndrome of multideficiencies in our body. During the aging process the hormone system is weakened (e.g., through a lack of insulin), many essential minerals are lost through natural or artificial processes, and antioxidant levels also decline. Therefore, in order to restore health and delay the aging processes it would be logical to focus on strengthening, supplementing, and regulating the natural functions of the human body.

Proper exercise should be an integral part of a diabetic treatment regimen. Dr. Young has an excellent review in this book on the rationale behind the medical significance of regular exercise on diabetes. He explains what constitutes the right kinds of exercise and links exercise to improving lymphatic circulation and cleansing—providing a particularly illuminating dimension for general readers.

This book will not be complete without Mrs. Shelley Redford Young's extensive recipes, which will certainly be appreciated, especially by those who cannot understand how anyone can actually live on a completely vegetarian diet. As one who has actually tasted and enjoyed the dishes prepared from these recipes, I believe that this section of the book can truly transform people's dietary habits into a way to take control of their diabetes and work toward an eventual cure.

Many years ago, when I first arrived at the National Institutes of Health to embark on my research career in the field of neurochemistry, a wise senior scientist advised me that a serious researcher should always dare to question and never blindly accept anything without thinking through and critically evaluating it. The importance of this inquisitive attitude was also pointed out by the great American physiologist Professor Walter B. Cannon in his book *The Way of an Investigator* in the early part of the twentieth century. Dr. Robert Young, a microbiologist and a true scientist in this inquisitive sense, boldly brings his independent research to bear on Louis Pasteur's germ theory of disease and ultimately rejects it, bringing into question what has been the bedrock of modern medicine for more than a century. Because of Pasteur's misguided doctrine, Dr. Young argues, diseases have been considered by modern medicine to be created solely by external insults. Thus the importance of the body's internal environment has totally been ignored. Modern therapeutic technologies have been designed in accordance to this thinking and are directed toward counteracting foreign attacks. Serious collateral damages to our normal body functions often occur as a result of this approach. Dr. Young rediscovered lost theories of great scientific minds from more than a century ago and developed his own New Biology, which is based on his understanding of acid–base balance. And so far the implemention of his theory has had a profound impact on the treatment of a wide array of diseases such as diabetes, cancers, chronic fatigue syndrome, obesity, urinary calculi, and more.

It is my belief that Dr. Young's theory, his therapeutic methodology, and his commitment to health care will continue to make history in years to come.

Chi C. Mao, M.D., Ph.D.
Chief Medical Officer
Select Specialty Hospitals—Houston
Houston, Texas

THE pH MIRACLE
FOR DIABETES

Chapter 1

Diabetes: The Epidemic—
and Working for the Cure

What lies behind us and what lies before us
are tiny matters compared to what lies within us.
—Ralph Waldo Emerson

My journey toward understanding the cause of—and demonstrating the cure for— Type 1 and Type 2 diabetes began in the Caribbean in the early 1990s. It was there, in Trinidad, Tobago, Grenada, and Barbados, that the proportions of the epidemic became clear to me. I knew, intellectually, that diabetes was the leading cause of death in the Caribbean (though the so-far-unanswered question *Why?* still nagged at me). But when I stood in front of an audience of a thousand islanders and asked (as part of a series of questions about common health issues) how many were challenged with diabetes, then watched half the people in the room raise their hands, I felt the enormity of the problem viscerally. I made up my mind right then to make it my mission to find the cause and the cure for diabetes.

It only took a few more questions about what the people I was addressing generally ate day to day to start seeing the roots of the problem. The answers quickly sketched out a diet consisting mainly of carbohydrates—sugars—heavy on fruit and root vegetables such as potatoes, along with chicken and some fish. That turned out to be the good news, such as it was. Although mainstream medicine would give those foods its seal of approval, as I later discovered it wasn't, in point of fact, a strong foundation. And it was now collapsing under the layers of sodas, pastries, candy, and American fast foods piled on top of it. As it turns out, my audience was consuming the perfect diet for creating diabetes. These people were enslaved to sugar, and it was killing them.

It took some years of study to understand and show it, but the solution was just as straightfoward as the problem. Shifting to a diet based on whole, natural foods, especially green vegetables, chosen to keep the body in pH balance (more about that coming right up!), could knock out diabetes and its many devastating health consequences, restoring a true island paradise free of such a plague.

It was, in fact, just the way of eating I'd come to recommend to my audience, for improved health in general. I just didn't realize at the time what an impact it could have on diabetes specifically.

I can't say I met with unanimous enthusiasm right off the bat. One man in the audience was probably speaking for many among the crowd when he stood up and said, "Doc, mon, we can't be eating the bush all the day long!" I wish I had then the data I have now about how "eating the bush all the day long" can save your life.

As it was, I assured him, as I'll assure you, that this is not just a healthful way to eat. It is also easy and delicious, thanks to the recipes and guidance my wife, Shelley, will provide. Give it a try, and you'll soon see for yourself how great you look and feel when you break the deadly hold your sugar-seeking taste buds have over you. It won't be long before you won't want to eat any other way. And, like most of the people I've worked with on this eating plan over the years, including forty participants in two organized studies, you'll be able to sit back and watch your blood sugar levels stabilize, to the point that you'll be able to cut back on or even eliminate any medication—including insulin.

The next chapter of the story unfolds in Houston in the spring of 1994. I was there for a research project on diabetes, and as part of it I interviewed a twenty-one-year-old woman with Type 1 diabetes.

She subsisted mostly on fast food and as many as fourteen cups of coffee a day. She didn't like vegetables, she said, and rarely ate them.

I proceeded as usual to analyze her blood using a technique I call live blood cell analysis. That is, I looked at her blood directly under a microscope—without using the fixatives usually used in making slides, which kills the cells. As I watched, stunned, a red blood cell turned into a bacterial cell. It moved through the blood plasma for a while, then, plain as day, turned back into a red blood cell.

All this was impossible according to everything I'd ever learned in twenty-plus years studying microbiology. I'd never have believed it if I hadn't seen it with my own two eyes. But the fact of what happened remained. In that one moment, everything I knew about human cells and bacteria cells was destroyed. My life as a microbiologist and nutritionist would never be the same. I'd happened on to the beginnings of a "New Biology." But I still had a few years ahead of me before I would understand that these cellular changes were actually to blame for the young woman's diabetes.

For two years, I thought I might be the only person on to this revolutionary view, and let me tell you, it was a lonely two years. I felt mine was a lone voice in the wilderness, and although I had a burning desire to share what I'd learned with the world, I couldn't see how I was going to get those who mattered most to listen, and understand that germs are the symptoms of cellular breakdown rather than the cause of any specific disease.

Then another microbiologist told me about the work Frenchman Antoine Bechamp had done in the late 1800s on "pleomorphism"— the many forms cells can take. I was ecstatic at the thought of other research that could help me understand my own work more deeply, not to mention relieved that I wasn't alone in my observations.

I quickly ran into a problem, however. Bechamp's work had been overtaken in his own time by his countryman Louis Pasteur's establishment of the germ theory of medicine, which still rules (if wrongly) today. I found a few references to Bechamp by combing through old or obscure sources, but I couldn't lay my hands on the originals. Plus, the originals, were they to be had, were entirely in

French. (I eventually unearthed the one book that had been translated into English: *The Blood and Its Third Anatomical Element.*)

My breakthrough moment came three years later. My wife, Shelley, and I were in Paris to celebrate our twenty-fifth wedding anniversary. There, in one of the most beautiful cities in the world, with the love of my life, I reveled in the romance of the City of Lights. But I was also intensely interested in something well off the typical tourist's beaten path: the University of Paris Medical Library, which I was guessing might house Bechamp's long-forgotten work.

As Shelley and I walked up the marble stairs at the library, I was thrilled at the prospect of what I might find. We were soon stopped by an attendant, however, who told us we could not enter the stacks without an official pass. My heart sank as my pleas that I had come all the way from America moved her not at all. Shelley and I used our sadly elementary French to try to persuade her for more than an hour before a passing Frenchman fluent in English rescued us, uttering whatever the magic phrases were to get us the aforementioned pass. This same kind gentleman then helped us locate Bechamp's work using a handwritten log of old books.

And then there I was, finally, marveling over Bechamp's twenty-seven published books and volumes of original research material like a little boy on Christmas morning. Here was the remarkable research of a great scientist, unearthed from the obscure archives in which it had been languishing for more than a hundred years. I had tears of joy in my eyes as I gently turned the pages, thunderstruck by the pictures Bechamp himself had sketched showing the biological transformation of a red blood cell to a bacterial cell over a century before my microscope revealed the same phenomenon to me in a young woman in Texas. Here was a man who had truly seen the magic of life. I had a lot to learn.

As I learned, and the theories of the New Biology coalesced in my mind, I started to see that diabetes is not in truth a disease of the pancreas or the insulin-producing beta cells, or an autoimmune response. Diabetes results, rather, from a disruption of the delicate pH balance (acid–base) in the fluids that surround the cells of the pancreas. Overacidity in the fluid allows cells to transform in negative ways, interfering with (among many other things) the way the body produces and uses insulin and sugar. On the other hand, with pH balance, the cells of the pancreas, insulin-producing beta cells, and glucagon-producing alpha cells could and would function in perfect harmony, and the phenomenon of diabetes could not occur. The mysteries of energy, health, fitness, and vitality are not revealed by focusing solely on the cells. The negative space, the fluids surrounding the cells, giving form and function to the cells, is at least as crucial. A cell is only as healthy as the fluids it is bathed in. I wrote about this extensively in my first book, *The pH Miracle*.

THE EPIDEMIC

Diabetes, a condition defined by high levels of sugar in the blood and the body's inability to make and/or use insulin, is a modern-day epidemic. There are an estimated seventeen to twenty million diabetics in the United States, somewhere between 6 and 8 percent of the population, with more than three-quarters of a million new cases each year. That's more than ever before in our history. Type 1 and Type 2 combine to be the third leading cause of death in the U.S., with more than three hundred thousand fatalities each year. Even those staggering numbers are relative small potatoes, however, when you consider that there are more than three hundred million diabetics worldwide, a figure that by some projections will double within a generation.

Women, people over sixty-five, African Americans, Hispanic people, Native Americans, Asian Americans, and Pacific Islanders are all at increased risk for Type 2 diabetes. Poor people are *three times* more likely to have it than middle- or high-income people. The American Diabetes Association (ADA) research shows that diabetes cost the United States $132 billion in medical care and lost wages in 2001 alone, up from $98 billion in 1997—as the epidemic spreads.

Diabetes can be severely debilitating and even fatal, due to side effects and complications including heart and kidney disease, blindness, nerve damage, and amputations. Tens of thousands of people lose their eyesight every year due to diabetes; it is the leading cause of blindness for people ages twenty-five through seventy-four. People with diabetes are about seven times as likely as people without it to become blind. That's according to a 1985 Emory University study, which also found diabetics to be twenty-five times more prone to gangrene (often leading to amputation), eleven times more likely to develop heart disease, and almost five and a half times more likely to have a stroke. Pregnancy diabetes increases the risk of premature delivery and even death of the baby. The bottom line of this tragedy is that the life expectancy of a person with diabetes is about a third shorter than the general population.

The vast majority—90 to 95 percent—of people with diabetes have the Type 2 variety. The vast majority—80 percent—of those with Type 2 are obese, which of course comes with its own huge set of negative health consequences. Every 1 mg increase in blood sugar represents a corresponding rise of 10 pounds, on average, in men and women both. It's no surprise that the recent increases in obesity in this country—more than half the country is now officially fat—has come hand in hand with increases in diabetes. About 1 percent of Americans had diabetes a century ago, but now we're looking at one in twelve people suffering from it. The rate of diabetes has increased by about half in the last decade alone, according to the Centers for Disease Control (CDC), and if current trends continue the ranks of those with diabetes can be expected to more than double in less than fifty years.

Type 2 diabetes used to be called adult-onset diabetes—as opposed to juvenile diabetes, sometimes called insulin-dependent, now known as Type 1. But that label has been dropped because it has become inaccurate: Diabetes is now the leading major chronic disease among children—and the one with the fastest rate of increase the world over. (Rates vary tremendously, however, from less than 1 child in 100,000 with Type 1 in Japan and parts of China to more than 28 per 100,000 in Finland, the world's leader in this regard. In the United States, almost 15 children in 100,000 are affected.) As the rate of obesity in children has risen dramatically in this country in recent years, so has the rate of Type 2 diabetes in children—where it used to be all but unknown. A 2003 CDC report projected that a third of American babies born in 2000 will develop diabetes.

Only about half of people with diabetes have received an official diagnosis, according to the Centers for Disease Control. The symptoms of diabetes often came on gradually, and with hallmarks you may not necessarily connect to blood sugar: general fatigue, light-headedness, dizziness, muddled thinking, forgetfulness, cold hands and feet, cloudy or blurred vision. So it may go undiagnosed for many years. If you don't know you have diabetes, you can't (or won't!) do anything to reverse it, or at least minimize the damage, so blood sugar levels should be part of your regular physical checkups at your doctor's office—it's one of the reasons you should have regular checkups, in fact.

As you see your doctor regularly, and perhaps obtain a diagnosis of diabetes, it is worth keeping in mind that the death rate from diabetes among doctors was reported to be 35 percent higher than that of the general population. That's what Bertrand E. Lowenstein, M.D., reported in his 1975 book *Diabetes*, where he placed the blame on conventional treatment methods, theorizing that doctors are more likely to be "good patients"—that is, to follow their treatment programs strictly—and so show the negative effects of those treatments more intensely.

Shelley and I witnessed the consequences of this in action in the Caribbean, watching many doctors with diabetes treating patients with diabetes. As the Good Book says, "If the blind lead the blind, both shall fall into the ditch" (Matthew 15:14). It was an eye-opening inspiration for us to find an alternative path. And I'm happy to be able to share it with you in this book.

THE pH MIRACLE

Mainstream medicine offers little real help with diabetes other than a lifetime of drugs and devastating potential side effects. In many cases, the best you can say of your options is that you can choose the lesser of the evils. Once you understand diabetes as a condition of the environment the cells are in, rather than a disease of the cells themselves, however, a new door opens to you, and you can use the simple, all-natural approach outlined in this book to help slow, stop, or even reverse diabetes and the damage it wreaks.

So the big question is how to provide the right environment for your cells. What lifestyle choices are optimum for maintaining pH balance in the body and eliminating illness and disease, including diabetes? I saw amazing results in people who simply learned to choose the best food, exercise, and supplements.

Denise's Story

I'm an overweight, Type 2 diabetic, and I've had high blood pressure for more than twenty years. That is, I was/did until I started using green drink with pH drops and eating more alkaline foods (though I haven't been able to go completely alkaline so far). In about two months, my blood sugar has gone from ranging between 153 and 228 to falling between 83 and 120. My blood pressure has normalized, and I have lost over 50 pounds! Now I know for myself why they call it the pH Miracle.

I started to check what happened to the blood of my clients as they adjusted their diets, and I saw that it came back into pH balance. As they corrected the acidity in their bodies by using the program in this book, I noted significant changes in specific health markers as well. I watched blood sugar, blood pressure, cholesterol count, and, last but not least, weight, all normalize. That quartet of diabetes, hypertension, hypercholesterolemia, and obesity occur so often together that mainstream medicine has dubbed the existence of all these diseases at once Syndrome X. And all of these diseases were disappearing in the patients on my program as the blood became more alkaline, and cells stabilized in healthy forms.

At first it was hard for me to believe that simple changes in what you eat and how you live could so dramatically impact the fluids of the body, which in turn had so much to do with the health of the cells. But as I saw it over and over again, I became convinced of the power of what I was seeing. By putting people on an aggressive pH Miracle diet that includes green foods, green drinks, moderate good fats, and low protein, I was seeing the reversal of Type 2 and even Type 1 diabetes. It was a real pH miracle.

Still, what I had so far amounted to no more than "anecdotal evidence" in the eyes of medical authorities. I knew in my heart that I had to do whatever was necessary to help others see what I was seeing. I couldn't let the current treatments of diabetes—which, by the way, don't offer real hope of a cure—go unchallenged. Too many lives depended on it. I knew there was a better way.

MY STUDIES

In 2002, I began a six-month controlled study on Type 1 and Type 2 diabetes, then ran another, for three months, in 2003. Both used the right alkaline food, aerobic exercise, and nutritional supplements. In *every case,* I found that the subjects who completed the program were able to decrease or discontinue their medications. That includes cutting their insulin intake by more than 50 percent, and in many cases eliminating insulin altogether, within just three months. The participants also lost weight, lowered their blood pressure, and reduced their total cholesterol.

I'd seen similar results in hundreds, if not thousands, of people I've worked with over the years—almost always with dramatic improvements in just the first seventy-two hours—but now for the first time I had a way of quantifying those results. For more than a decade, I'd watched as people going on the program normalized their blood sugars, and seen several doctors throughout the country begin to recommend the program to their patients (or even use it themselves!), but this more rigorous confirmation was powerful. I'm now working with the University of Miami to set up another, larger controlled study, and look forward to even more convincing data.

Both of my studies began with a two-week liquid feast. The first study followed this with one month of a strict alkaline diet, then the remainder of the total six months on a diet that was 80 percent alkaline. The second study lasted a total of only three months, all of which was on the strict diet. Participants in both followed essentially the same plan outlined in this book, avoiding all dairy, sweets, grains, and meat (except fish), as well as most fruits, and were encouraged to eat liberal amounts of good fats and oils. They used green drinks with pH drops and a program of supplements, again much the same as the one you'll see detailed later in this book—an herbal multivitamin, multimineral supplement; sprouted soy powder; essential fatty acids (EFAs); chromium and vanadium; the coenzyme supplement always known by its initials, NADP; an herbal cleanser (a mild laxative); an adrenal support formula; a pancreas support formula; and, in the second study, clay.

People in the study reported daily in online computer logs about everything they ate, the supplements they took, how much insulin or other medication they took and when, morning and evening blood sugar readings, and weight; they reported weekly on blood pressure. We held weekly conference calls so I could answer any questions they had, and we set up an e-mailing system where participants exchanged advice, support—and recipes.

A total of twenty people completed one or the other of the studies, nine with Type 1 and eleven with Type 2 diabetes. (Ten others dropped out along the way, mostly because they could not handle the diet in the second study.) The table that follows gives an overview of the specific results.

Everyone who finished the study reduced or eliminated their medication. The Type 2 diabetics averaged a 96 percent reduction in their insulin or other diabetic medications, and the Type 1 people reduced insulin an average of 81 percent. People with Type 2 had even greater success than those with Type 1, in general, although the Type 1 results are impressive nonetheless. With the stricter diet in the second study, Type 1 diabetics experienced better control of their blood sugar than those in the first study did. All participants completing either study maintained normal blood sugars. And everyone lost weight—an average of 32 pounds after twelve weeks.

STUDY RESULTS

	Type (1 or 2)	Beginning Weight (pounds)	Weight After 12 Weeks (pounds)	Weight Loss (pounds)	Lowest Sugar Levels at Start of Program, with *Meds* (mg/dl)	Highest Sugar Levels at Start of Program, with *Meds* (mg/dl)	Lowest Sugar Levels After 12 Weeks on Program, Without (or with Reduced) Meds (mg/dl)	Highest Sugar Levels After 12 Weeks on Program, Without (or with Reduced) Meds (mg/dl)
Male, 48	1	244	174	70	30	500	68 (insulin reduced 70%)	180
Female, 10	1	85	80	5	77	300	100 (insulin reduced 50%)	126
Female, 50	1	140	118	22	27	390	60 (insulin reduced 85%)	220
Female, 38	1	200	130	70	199	386	100	140
Female, 38	1	345	255	90	50	270	70	120
Male, 29	1	200	145	55	20	300	60 (insulin reduced 80%)	170
Male, 36	1	115	109	6	40	400+	64 (insulin reduced 80%)	127
Male, 53	1	112	108	4	60	123	70	114
Male, 32	1	115	109	6	65	129	72 (insulin reduced 65%)	111

(continued)

	Type (1 or 2)	Beginning Weight (pounds)	Weight After 12 Weeks (pounds)	Weight Loss (pounds)	Lowest Sugar Levels at Start of Program, with *Meds* (mg/dl)	Highest Sugar Levels at Start of Program, with *Meds* (mg/dl)	Lowest Sugar Levels After 12 Weeks on Program, Without (or with Reduced) Meds (mg/dl)	Highest Sugar Levels After 12 Weeks on Program, Without (or with Reduced) Meds (mg/dl)
Female, 55	2	340	294	48	35	215	66	115
Female, 38	2	265	232	34	40	125	64	110
Male, 58	2	275	248	27	40	278	48	154
Male, 61	2	245	213	32	48	205	76	133
Female, 36	2	210	177	33	50	230	60	98
Male, 53	2	267	233	34	45	300	62	105
Female, 55	2	307	268	39	50	127	73	110
Female, 34	2	180	155	25	41	262	70	127
Male, 32	2	150	150	0	55	339	68	127
Male, 52	2	274	222	52	60	160	80	108
Male, 59	2	200	196	4	59	220	80 (insulin reduced 50%)	140

Stephen's Story

I was twenty-one years old, I had played college football and was extremely healthy—and I had just been diagnosed with Type 1 diabetes. I resisted my fiancée's pleadings to seek holistic treatment, determined to follow my conventional doctor's orders; after all, he knew best. Well, six doctors and twenty-seven years later, diabetes was severely taxing my tired, overweight body. I had developed kidney problems and high blood pressure, and spent five days in intensive care with blood sugars over 1,100.

But this was not the worst of it. That came this year, when my nine-year-old daughter was diagnosed with Type 1 diabetes. Refusing to accept this "diabetic death sentence" for Molly, and having never stopped praying for my complete healing, my wife began searching for alternatives. She soon found the pH Miracle plan, and we promptly put the principles into practice, beginning with a liquid feast, coupled with supplements, and moving into an alkaline diet. My daughter and I regularly monitored our blood sugar and pH levels.

The results have been dramatic. Molly's need for insulin has been systematically reduced, and she goes some days with no insulin at all. Likewise, I have reduced my insulin intake by over half. I also lost 51 pounds and was able to stop taking high blood pressure medication—within the first six weeks!

This has been a great blessing for my whole family. I never imagined a greater joy than reclaiming my own health, but knowing my daughter will never suffer what I have is it.

If that's not a pH miracle, I don't know what is. The beauty of it is, it isn't really a miracle at all. It may seem like one when all you've ever heard about diabetes is that there is no cure, that you'll need those injections, or that medication, forever—and that even then, there aren't many happy endings. But there's no mystery to this; not once you know how to get your body back in pH balance. You can have the same results in your own life as the participants in my studies did, simply by following the plan in this book. It's not a substitute for medical care, and you'll still need to work closely with your doctor. But this way, rather than a potential lifetime sentence of ill health, in just twelve weeks you'll be well on your way to experiencing full health and wellness—without the high doses of medication most diabetes patients use. *Your* journey to the cure has just begun.

Chapter 2

What Is Diabetes?

Physicians of the utmost fame
Were called at once; but when they came
They answered, as they took their fees
"There is no cure for this disease."
—HILAIRE BELLOC (1870–1953)

Diabetes is a Greek word meaning "to siphon or pass through." And, indeed, a hallmark of diabetes is excessive urination (and the resulting all but unquenchable thirst) as the body tries desperately to get rid of excess sugar and maintain a pH balance. Second-century Greek physician Aretaeus observed that his patients' bodies appeared to "melt down" into urine. He echoed the words of Egyptian Third Dynasty physician Hesy-ra, who wrote in about 1550 B.C. that diabetes caused a "melting down"—and that the resulting urine attracted ants because of its high sugar content. By the eighteenth century, doctors added *mellitus* to the name of the diagnosis, which is Latin referring to honey or a sweet taste. It was as if a person with diabetes mellitus was melting into sugar. The diagnosis of diabetes was frequently confirmed by "water tasters," who detected sugar in the urine by its sweet taste. Folk wisdom has dictated an at-home test for diabetes: Spill urine on newspaper and let it dry; the results are shiny with sugar crystals in people who have diabetes.

In this way, people with diabetes are not unlike bananas. Stay with me for a minute here. We all know that bananas get sweeter the older they get. As they age or ripen, bananas do indeed increase in sugar content—or rather, their cells release their sugars as they begin to break down. The bananas soften, too, of course: They are melting into sugar. Or, you might say, rotting. It is interesting to note that the black spots on the surface of an overripe banana's skin are the acids from the breakdown of the banana's cells. This is the same phenomenon that happens to all plant and animal cells, including human cells. As they age (ripen, rot), they disorganize and "melt into sugar." This whole process might be good news for fans of banana bread just like my mom used to make, but there is no upside in humans.

DOCTORS AND DIABETES

No doubt your doctor didn't explain diabetes to you in quite that way. There, you probably heard that diabetes is caused by a partial or total lack of the hormone insulin in the body, resulting in excessively high levels of glucose (sugar) in the blood. But what really causes a serious degenerative disease such as diabetes? I mean *really* causes it; phrases such as *high blood sugar* or *low insulin* describe the condition but don't explain it. What causes the body to be insufficiently or excessively supplied with those things? And why is it that some people develop diabetes while others under similar conditions do not?

As it circulates through the body, blood always carries a certain amount of sugar to provide fuel for the cells. Getting sugar into the cells requires insulin, which is produced in the pancreas by what are called beta cells. Normally, the pancreas produces just enough insulin to handle the body's needs from moment to moment. In diabetes, however, the insulin is either absent, in short supply, or unable to perform its job effectively. Sugar that cannot get into the cells accumulates in the bloodstream.

TYPE 1 AND TYPE 2 DIABETES

Doctors consider diabetes as having two distinct forms. In Type 1, or insulin-dependent diabetes mellitus (IDDM), the beta cells of the pancreas do not produce sufficient amounts of insulin. People in this group must take insulin injections daily to stay alive. Type 1 diabetes used to be known as juvenile diabetes because it typically first appears in children and young adults. This is the most serious type of diabetes, and it accounts for 5 to 10 percent of all cases.

Type 2 diabetes—non-insulin-dependent diabetes mellitus (NIDDM)—is far more common, but less drastic. It, too, can be deadly, however, and certainly wreaks havoc with your quality of life. In Type 2, the beta cells are making insulin, but the body isn't using it effectively. This condition is referred to as insulin resistance. People with Type 2 diabetes do not usually require insulin injections, though they may if they fail to control their blood sugar levels over the long run. Many people with Type 2 diabetes use a range of oral medications to control their blood sugar levels. With insulin resistance, in an attempt to handle sugar in the blood the pancreas pumps out ever more insulin that the body doesn't respond to, and the beta cells can eventually give up altogether and stop making the hormone, or make hardly enough to make a difference.

The big problem with diabetes, whether Type 1 or Type 2, isn't even the condition itself, but the long list of devastating side effects that come with it. Diabetes puts you on a path toward heart disease, kidney failure, nerve damage, blindness, disability, and even death.

About 80 percent of people with Type 2 diabetes are overweight. Historically, Type 2 was typically diagnosed in people over the age of forty. One of the multiple tragedies of the recent explosion in the rate of obesity in children is that Type 2 diabetes is now commonly turning up even in young children. It appears that the typical American lifestyle has created diabetes in epidemic proportions across age groups.

Tracy's Story

My daughter Tracy was just twenty when she was diagnosed with Type 1 diabetes and prescribed 130 units a day of insulin, which the doctor said she would need for the rest of her life. She was also told she had high blood pressure, high cholesterol, and high triglycerides, and she was given medications for all those conditions as well. Three years later, she became deathly ill, and was eventually diagnosed with fibromyalgia and chronic fatigue syndrome. She was totally disabled, unable to work or drive. She couldn't sleep, and walking a few feet was a struggle.

As a mother, it was very painful to see such a young, vibrant, joyful person suffering in such a manner, with no apparent hope for recovery. But through it all, Tracy remained optimistic and cheerful. Truly, she is the bravest person I know.

Over the last seven years, Tracy saw more than twenty highly specialized doctors, none of whom offered much hope for any real relief. Tracy refused to accept this way of life, but gave up on getting help through conventional medicine. She went on an odyssey of alternative treatments, determined to find a cure for herself. Finally she found what we affectionately call "Miracle Water"—a green drink with pH drops—which she started taking, along with supplements to support the pancreas, adrenals, and kidneys, as well as eating an alkaline diet.

In just five weeks, Tracy was once again an energetic young woman, brimming with vitality. She is off all her medications, including the four shots of 35 to 40 units of insulin she'd been taking each day for more than seven years. She lost over 20 pounds, and her recent blood work was the best it had ever been, with blood sugars under 100.

Sadly, my husband, Brian, was soon thereafter diagnosed with Type 2 diabetes, with blood sugars in excess of 350. He began drinking Miracle Water and taking supplements to support the pancreas. With his newfound energy, he began to exercise regularly. Today, his fasting blood glucose level is normal (93)!

I was so impressed, inspired, and awed with my daughter's and husband's recoveries from diabetes and related symptoms that I started using the green drink with pH drops myself, as well as eating right and, with the energy I soon found I had, exercising. I had a blood test several weeks after starting. In going over the results with me, my doctor told me I was very healthy—for a twenty-nine-year-old woman! (Ha, ha.) Plus, this is the easiest way to lose weight I've ever experienced—I dropped an extra 20 pounds in just thirty days. Now Brian and Tracy aren't the only ones who look and feel great!

GESTATIONAL DIABETES

One other common type of diabetes is gestational diabetes, or diabetes occurring during pregnancy in women who haven't had diabetes before. Gestational diabetes has the same risk factors and symptoms as Type 2 diabetes, although its potential for troublemaking is, by its nature, double: trouble for the mother and trouble for the baby. Make that quadruple trouble, because you face all the problems of Type 2 diabetes in general, plus special problems stemming from being diabetic while pregnant.

A study of twenty-three thousand pregnant, obese women with Type 2 diabetes showed they are three times as likely as nondiabetic pregnant women of normal weight to have babies with birth defects—seven times as likely to have a baby with a craniofacial defect such as cleft palate or abnormal limb development. Nearly 6 percent of babies born to women with Type 2 diabetes have major defects.

Uncontrolled gestational diabetes increases the risk for a difficult delivery or C-section, as well as the chances of the baby being born with dangerously low blood sugar, jaundice, or breathing problems.

Babies of moms with gestational diabetes tend to weigh much more than normal, and that creates special health problems, including potential damage to their shoulders during birth. These babies have excess insulin, which puts them at higher risk of developing obesity and Type 2 diabetes themselves. Diabetes that starts during pregnancy usually goes away after the baby is born, but you'll still be at increased risk of developing Type 2 diabetes later in your life.

MEASURING BLOOD SUGAR LEVELS

Normal blood sugars, tested after you've fasted for at least eight hours, should be 110 mg/dl or less. (If tested *not* on an empty stomach, then it should be 140 mg/dl or less.) If your levels are between 110 and 126 fasting (or between 140 and 200 not fasting), that's called impaired glucose tolerance (GLT) and is considered prediabetes. Higher than those numbers, and you officially have diabetes. To confirm a diagnosis, your doctor may give you a glucose tolerance test, drawing your blood two hours after you've had a certain amount of sugar-water solution to drink. If your blood sugar level then is 200 mg/dl or above, you're diabetic.

CAUSES OF DIABETES

According to traditional medical science, the cause of diabetes is something of a mystery. A leading theory is that Type 1 is an autoimmune disorder in which white blood cells attack and destroy the insulin-producing beta cells in the pancreas as if they were threatening invaders. The roots of Type 2 diabetes are more fully mapped out, and obesity is at the epicenter. Just what it is about carrying around extra weight that makes the body's production and use of insulin go haywire isn't clearly understood, though. Indeed, this is still a chicken-and-egg question: Does obesity cause diabetes, or does diabetes bring on obesity?

Looking at this through the lens of New Biology, however, it becomes clear that diabetes is *not* a disease of the pancreas or the beta cells therein. Rather, it is the result of a pH imbalance in the fluids of the body—systemic acidosis—that interferes with the optimum functioning of the cells they surround. Beta cells surrounded by acids do not or cannot produce sufficient insulin. Acids destroy insulin receptor sites on the cellular membrane so body cells cannot properly use the hormone. Diabetic symptoms—which can include frequent urination, extreme thirst, ravenous hunger, weight loss, extreme fatigue, muscle wasting, and life-threatening ketoacidosis—are all a result of the body attempting to regain or maintain the delicate pH balance of the blood and tissues.

THE NEW BIOLOGY

I more thoroughly explain the principles of the New Biology in our previous book, *The pH Miracle,* and if you want to really understand more of the science of the theory you can review it there. For our purposes in this book, I just want to briefly review the key points. Then we'll get on, without any further delay, to what you can do to free yourself from the grip of diabetes.

The one indicator most crucial to your health is not your blood sugar level—or your weight, blood pressure, cholesterol, or anything else—but the pH of your blood. That is, how acidic or alkaline (basic) it is. The pH scale runs from 1.0 (most acidic) to 14.0 (most alkaline), with 7.0 being neutral. Just as your body strictly maintains its temperature, it will do anything and everything it can to keep the blood in a very narrow pH range—a mildly alkaline 7.365 pH. (Some bodily systems, notably the stomach and colon, are rightly acidic, though it is all too easy for them to swing too far in that direction.) The pH level of the blood and other bodily fluids and tissues affects every single cell. The whole metabolic process depends on alkalinity as well—overacidity is what keeps you fat. Just about every negative symptom you can think of—not least of which is the cluster of symptoms surrounding diabetes—happens when the body has to go to desperate extremes in an attempt to maintain its pH.

One of the potentially most devastating effects of an acidic environment in your body is the cozy home that this makes for yeast, fungi, mold, bacteria, and viruses, known collectively as microforms. While many of these live benignly or beneficially in a healthy body by design, nasty ones thrive in an acidic environment, and even the nice guys can overgrow enough to become harmful. And then we get a triple whammy: Not only can the microforms themselves be dangerous, but they can also create poisonous (acidic) excretions, exotoxins and mycotoxins, which they do as they digest—or ferment—the energy sources our bodies would otherwise use themselves, and release those acids into the bloodstream.

This is where Bechamp's work fits in. What he discovered, and what I've seen so many times in my own microscope, is that harmful microforms *can come from our own cells*. I'll give you one guess as to what kind of environment must exist for this to happen. That's right: acid. Not to mention the fact that external microforms (germs) can only contribute to illness when they land in such an environment.

As Bechamp described so many years ago, our bodies, like all living things, contain what are called microzymas living independently in cells and body fluids. These can and do evolve into more complex forms—all cells evolve from them in the first place. And in some environments, microzymas evolve into bacteria and fungi. Harmful microforms can also de-evolve back to microzymas, a much happier state of affairs that, no surprise, depends on a healthy (nonacidic) environment. As microforms evolve, they change form and function (depending on the environment), which I call pleomorphism. Harmful pleomorphic organisms do not, and cannot, evolve in healthy (alkaline) surroundings. This is the true nature of matter, and the way it organizes and disorganizes. Physical or even emotional disturbances can cause disorganization, or de-evolution, which in turn acidifies the environment further still, creating a vicious cycle.

In this way of looking at things, there is only one sickness (overacidification) and one cure (restoring alkalinity). Acidity in different tissues of the body shows up with different sets of symptoms, which have had various disease labels slapped on them by mainstream medical science.

When the acidity is in the pancreas, diabetes is the result. But all these problems trace back to the same thing, though science has focused too much on the trees to be able to see this forest. The beauty of seeing that whole forest at last is that the pathway running through it to good health for each and every one of us becomes clear and attainable.

ARE YOU ACIDIC?

You can check the pH level of your own blood at home with simple paper pH strips, available at many pharmacies, or with a battery-operated pH electron meter, available from health catalogs (see the resources section). The strips are pretty inexpensive, and test the pH of your saliva or urine; I recommend testing your urine first thing in the morning, after you've fasted overnight, for the most accurate results. The strips change color to indicate acid or base, and are lighter or darker depending on the intensity of the reading. They come with a color chart to help you translate the color into a number.

The meters are also best used to test your urine first thing in the morning, though they can be used to test saliva as well. They provide clear, accurate results, but can be hard to find and are expensive, running into the hundreds of dollars.

Your doctor can also do a blood pH test for you. The ideal blood pH is 7.365, though the American medical establishment accepts 7.4, so you should be sure you get your exact result, rather than just a report of "normal."

THE NEW BIOLOGY OF DIABETES

Your body maintains its pH balance by drawing on stores of alkaline substances—mainly minerals such as sodium, potassium, calcium, and magnesium. Fighting excessive acidity overwhelms those stores (and/or poor nutrition means inadequate stores in the first place), and your body draws the substances from where your body is trying to put them to good use by taking calcium from the bones, for example, or magnesium from muscles. Naturally, this leaves those areas weakened; the pancreas is one of the vulnerable spots.

In addition, when the blood is overly acid, it begins to unload the excess acids into the body's tissues, storing them in protective fat in the breasts, hips, belly, and even in the brain, heart—and pancreas. Overly acidic blood stimulates the immune system to try to get rid of the overload, and this can quickly overtax your immune defenses, once again leaving you vulnerable to diabetes (among many other things).

All body cells—including those famous beta cells—must continually break down and renew themselves to stay hearty. In a healthy, alkaline environment, microforms are there to take care of the recycling, so to speak. They clean up the normal waste products of cellular breakdown and metabolism so our bodies won't become toxic waste dumps. All bets are off in an acidic environment, however. The good microforms get overwhelmed and can't process all the waste they are swimming in; they then start multiplying like crazy and producing copious quantities of toxic waste of their own. When those toxins aren't eliminated, or aren't eliminated quickly or completely enough, the acid is retained in the blood and tissues, tending to localize at weak parts of the body. When acid localizes to the pancreas, diabetes results. All the symptoms of diabetes come back to this same root.

In a healthy body, microzymes help renew the beta cells, but if you fall out of alkaline balance, breakdown/fermentation/aging/rotting eventually takes over. Then beta cells die or disorganize or de-evolve, increasing acidity without the renewal part of the natural cycle to even things out. The acidic environment prematurely signals the microzymas that the organism is out of balance. They then change function and form, becoming viruses, bacteria, yeasts, or molds with ever-more-vigorous cellular breakdown capabilities. If alkalinity is not soon restored, disease, including diabetes, takes hold. But without acidosis, there can be no sickness or disease— there can be no diabetes.

Kevin's Story

I've had Type 1 diabetes for thirty-three years, since the age of three. Before I started on this plan, my blood sugar levels often ran between 300 and 400 or more. But now with green drink, supplements, and an alkaline diet, I've got my diabetes under control. After all these years, I no longer need to take any insulin of any kind—and my blood sugars have evened out more than ever before, normally falling between 64 and 127. My Type 1 diabetcs is almost eliminated!

A DANGEROUS GAME

Current medical science theorizes that diabetes may be genetic; scientists have pinpointed certain proteins in certain cells that scem to predispose the people who have them to getting Type 1 diabetes. But get this: Even though about 25 percent of American children are predisposed in this way, fewer than 1 percent of this group actually develops the disease. Also, when one identical twin has the disease, only half of the time does the other twin have it as well. (For genetic conditions, you'd expect a 100 percent match in identical twins.)

Those proteins show up with the same frequency pretty much wherever you go, but the prevalence of diabetes varies widely in different places around the world. Less than 1 in 100,000 Japanese are affected, compared to 9 in the United States and more than 28 in Finland (which has the unfortunate distinction of being the country with the highest rate in the world today). Furthermore, in some places around the world, rates of the disease have been increasing far more steeply than could be explained by heredity. Consider, for example, the shocking 50 percent increase in diabetes in children under ten years of age over the last twenty years in Finland.

Diabetes turns out to be a dangerous game, not unlike Russian roulette. The genetic bullet only does damage if the lifestyle triggers are pulled. Your genes themselves do not cause diabetes, but living out of balance can unleash their potential to harm. Later chapters look more in depth at a variety of causes of unstable blood sugar, including carbohydrates, alcohol, caffeine, low-fat diets, anaerobic exercise, psychological stress, fear or anger, and lack of certain nutrients. All these things cause excess acidity, and excess acidity, especially from an unhealthy diet, leads to the pancreas increasing the amount of insulin it releases, which stresses the pancreas, which eventually burns out. Voilà: diabetes.

Understanding and interrupting this cycle will improve both the quality and the quantity of your life, because the right path becomes compellingly obvious: Stay in pH balance. As soon as acidity is controlled, the symptoms disappear. Even an organ put through innumerable crises—as with the pancreas in uncontrolled diabetes—will be rejuvenated once the true underlying cause of the problem is eliminated. As we like to say around here: Get off your fat acid, and go to health!

Chapter 3

The Many Faces of Type 1 and Type 2 Diabetes

*What we already know is a great hindrance
in discovering the unknown.*
—CLAUDE BERNARD, FRENCH PHYSIOLOGIST (1813–1878)

There's a long, long list of symptoms associated with diabetes. The most familiar may be disturbed blood sugar levels, but that's just the beginning. In fact, blood sugar levels may be off for some time before they are caught—often only when some of these other symptoms are being investigated. The sooner you stabilize your blood sugar levels—preventing the many negative symptoms from developing—the better. This chapter walks you through the many signs your body may be sending you that all is not right, so that you may answer that call swiftly if it comes. But our fondest wish is that for you this chapter will be nothing more than a field guide to a world you'll never enter. I hope it will stir all readers' resolve to eat right in order to power their bodies for good health.

HYPERGLYCEMIA AND HYPOGLYCEMIA

Among the beginning symptoms of excess acidity leading toward diabetes are hypoglycemia (low blood sugar) and hyperglycemia (high blood sugar). The two may seem to be opposites, but really they are two sides of the same coin. Both stem from sugar addiction and the acid environment sugar creates in the body.

Hyperglycemia indicates an obvious problem with insulin production or use—it simply isn't there, or isn't doing its job (handling sugar). Low blood sugar, which is very common, actually indicates overblown insulin production—insulin working overtime.

The pancreas produces two hormones to regulate blood sugar: insulin, which is supposed to make sure blood sugar levels don't get too high, and glucagon, which keeps them from dropping too low. Insulin helps clear sugar from the bloodstream by helping transport it across cell membranes into the cells to be used to produce energy. In addition, insulin acts on the liver to convert sugar into glycogen and fat for storage. Glucagon sends a message to the liver and then to the muscles to convert stored carbohydrates (glycogen) back into sugar (glucose); to convert other nutrients, such as amino acids, into glucose; and to release the sugar into the bloodstream.

Your body responds to the low blood sugar as you would respond to the fuel light coming on in your car: You fill it up as soon as you can with more of the same. Being called on to process more and more sugar creates such stress on the pancreas that it will eventually burn out and give up making insulin altogether. The symptoms of low or high blood sugar can be unpleasant enough on their own (see the box), but more serious still is the fact that this seesawing from low to high blood sugar sets the stage for full-blown diabetes.

That's as much as your doctor is likely to explain to you. The deeper explanation of New Biology takes into account that negative microforms such as bacteria and especially yeast have a ferocious appetite for sugar. As they ferment your blood sugar, your blood sugar naturally drops, and you are left with their acidic waste products. The more acidic the environment, the more those nasty little things love it, and they multiply like crazy: You've entered another vicious cycle. And they are hungry! It isn't so much *you* craving all

SYMPTOMS OF LOW BLOOD SUGAR*

- Weakness
- Fatigue
- Rapid heartbeat
- Shakiness
- Dizziness
- Sweating
- Hunger
- Headache
- Impaired vision; double vision
- Loss of coordination
- Loss of concentration
- Muddled thinking
- Nausea
- Forgetfulness
- Nightmares
- Irritability
- Anger
- Pale skin color
- Moodiness
- Clumsiness or jerkiness
- Confusion
- Difficulty paying attention
- Tingling sensations around the mouth
- Cold hands and feet
- Convulsions
- Inability to wake up; coma

* Symptoms become more severe the lower your blood sugar gets.

SYMPTOMS OF HIGH BLOOD SUGAR

- Extreme thirst
- Frequent urination
- Confusion
- Sleepiness
- Dry skin
- Inability to perspire
- Blurred vision
- Hunger
- Diabetic coma or ketoacidosis
- Shortness of breath
- Nausea
- Vomiting
- Dry mouth
- Extreme fatigue and tiredness

that sugar, it's the yeast and bacteria that you are playing host to. Furthermore, moving glycogen from the muscles to the blood comes at a cost: The process increases acidity, and encourages the growth of yeast.

Doctors use, as a rule of thumb, blood sugar levels of 60 mg/dl as the borderline for normal. With levels there or lower, they'd expect to see signs and symptoms of hypoglycemia. Your body doesn't function very well when you have too little glucose (sugar) in your blood. Your muscles need the energy that glucose provides to do their work, and with insufficient levels, you'll feel weak, tired, and uncoordinated, and may experience muscle soreness, irritation, and inflammation. Your brain needs glucose to run the rest of your body. Not to mention to run itself, providing all your intellectual processes. Without enough sugar, you won't think clearly, concentrate well, or remember reliably. You may know the right thing to do, but be unable to do it.

Sam's Story

I'm sixty-two, and have been on oral medications for Type 2 diabetes for five years. In just four weeks taking green drinks and eating an alkaline diet, I have been able to reduce my doses between 50 and 75 percent—while getting the best blood sugar levels I've ever had. Plus, I've lost 7 pounds, and counting. And to think, I was told this was an incurable, increasingly debilitating condition!

INSULIN RESISTANCE

Hypoglycemia can lead to hyperglycemia from sugar cravings and glycogen conversions, and these in turn can lead to hyperinsulinemia (too much insulin), then insulin resistance—and from there the next step is full-blown Type 2 diabetes. Over time, the alternating surges of sugar and insulin, and the acid created from the fermentation of the excess sugars, damage the receptor sites for glucose on the surface of the cells. Those cells can't receive the glucose they need for energy, the sugar is left in the bloodstream, and more and more insulin is released. The body no longer responds properly to the insulin—it can't complete its mission of transporting sugar to the cells that could use it. Meanwhile, the body grows ever more acidic, and negative microforms are more and more at home, and set about creating even more acid.

WHAT TO DO WHEN YOU HAVE LOW BLOOD SUGAR

Following the pH Miracle plan will free you from low blood sugar and its ill effects. You may still have to deal with an episode in the meantime. No doubt you have differing instructions from your doctor, but they aren't compatible with the pH Miracle plan. Eating a candy bar or having a glass of apple juice or something else to provide a big jolt of sugar may work in the short term—you'll have a very temporary burst of energy replacing that low blood sugar fatigue—but the longer-term effect will be to increase acids from bacteria or yeast fermentation, buying you a ticket on the same old merry-go-round. Here are some equally good solutions that won't contribute to acidity:

- Drink a glass of fresh almond milk.
- Snack on a carrot or beet.
- Eat a bowl of tomatoes with avocado.
- Drink a liter of green drink.

> ## WHAT TO DO WHEN YOU
> ## HAVE HIGH BLOOD SUGAR
>
> Following the pH Miracle plan, you should eliminate acute
> episodes of hyperglycemia. If you have any of the serious
> symptoms detailed above, you need to address them immedi-
> ately. Rehydrate by drinking large volumes of green drink,
> 1 liter for every 30 pounds of your body weight. Take chromium,
> which helps bind insulin and glucose to take sugar into the cell
> for use as an energy source.

SYMPTOMS AND SIGNS

Beyond the signs of low or high blood sugar as detailed above, there
are a host of other potential problems that come along with a diagnosis of diabetes. If the earlier side effects lists don't promise enough
misery to make you determined to maintain your sugar at healthy
levels, how about serious cardiovascular complications, nerve or kidney damage, blindness or other vision problems, and elevated risk of
needing a limb amputated? All these and more can be traced back to
not just unhealthy blood sugar levels, but also overacidity of the
body. Put them all together and what you have is premature aging
as, not to put too fine a point on it, our bodies rot.

Heart

Let's start with the heart. Having diabetes doubles or quadruples
your chance of having heart-related problems including heart
attack, atherosclerosis, angina, stroke, high blood pressure, high
triglycerides, and high cholesterol. The body protects itself from
excess acids (from excess sugars)—which could bore holes in blood

vessels—by binding them with fats and minerals. But those fats build up in the blood vessels and heart, causing atherosclerosis, angina, heart attack, and stroke. Your heart then has to work harder to move blood to and from itself, pushing the same volume of blood through narrowed blood vessels, meaning elevated blood pressure. (Nearly 60 percent of people with high blood pressure are diabetic.) Damaged, weakened heart and blood vessels can also cause your blood pressure to spike when you rise quickly from a seated position, leaving you feeling light-headed or dizzy. The same may happen when you've been standing for long periods of time.

Your body also elevates LDL cholesterol to bind acids, and triglycerides to help protect itself from excess acids from the fermentation of excess sugar. The so-called bad cholesterol (LDL) is literally saving your life from excess acidity in the short term—at the cost of risking your life through heart problems over the long term.

Acids are very sticky and can cause cells to stick together, causing circulation problems such as intermittent claudication (pain or numbness in lower limbs while walking) and oxygen deprivation, which leads to cold hands and feet, muddled thinking, forgetfulness and memory loss, light-headedness, dizziness, and even dementia. Congestive heart failure can be traced to sugars turning to acids and turning your heart muscles to mush.

Vision

Diabetic retinopathy is the name given to damage to the vessels supplying blood to the retina. It can cause blindness. In fact, diabetes is the leading cause of new blindness. Many vision problems are increased in people with diabetes, including glaucoma (pressure on the eye restricting blood to the optic nerve) and cataracts (calcifications on the eye causing loss of vision acuity; the body uses calcium to neutralize excess acids), both of which are about one and a half times more common in those with diabetes. Diabetes is also associated with an increase in rates of macular edema (loss of vision acuity) and neo-vascularization (hemorrhagic glaucoma), again thanks to excess acidity.

Kidney

Within fifteen years, 20 percent of people with diabetes will develop kidney disease, which can lead to end-stage renal disease or kidney failure. The kidneys flat-out give up and shut down after all that time dealing with eliminating sugar-created acids.

Nerves

Sixty to 70 percent of people with diabetes have nervous system damage that can create a wide range of symptoms, including tingling, burning, numbness, loss of sensitivity to heat and cold, and sharp stabbing pains or "pins and needles," especially in the hands and feet, and ranging up to impaired digestion, excessive sweating, erectile dysfunction, and interference with blood pressure and heartbeat. Foot drop is one example, a condition in which the foot cannot be raised properly due to damage to the nerves that supply the foot. Incontinence (poor bladder control) is another. It results when nerves to the bladder are damaged, leading to bladder distention, leaking, and/or difficulty emptying the bladder, which in turn increases the incidence of urinary tract infections.

Amputation

Over sixty-seven thousand legs are amputated each year in the United States due to diabetes-related problems; more than half could be prevented with early detection and correct lifestyle and diet. The problem is especially acute among African Americans and Native Americans, who are up to four times more likely than the general population to have diabetes. Poor circulation is an underlying cause, and it surfaces first as foot ulcers, which get infected, then produce gangrene (molding, rotting tissue treated by surgical removal).

Obesity

Rather than burning body fat off, in a crisis, trying desperately to preserve itself, the body hoards all fat and uses it to park as much acid as it can safely away from the organs that sustain life.

Gastrointestinal Problems

Gastrointestinal upset is common in people with diabetes, whether nausea, vomiting, constipation, or diarrhea. All of these can slow the action of the stomach or gut muscles, leading to inefficient emptying of the digestive tract. Diabetic gastroparesis is when the stomach empties too slowly into the small intestine because the nerves that control the pace have been damaged. For people who take insulin before a meal, that can mean their blood sugar falls before the food has a chance to be absorbed.

Sexual Dysfunction

More than half of all men over fifty who have diabetes also experience impotence; men with diabetes develop impotence ten to fifteen years earlier, on average, than healthy men. Over a third of women with diabetes experience diminished sexual function of some kind, including reduced sensitivity to touch due to nerve damage, vaginal dryness, and decreased desire. Sexual function and desire are products of the autonomic nervous system, which can be paralyzed by overacidity.

Osteoporosis

The body draws calcium from the bones to neutralize acids and maintain the delicate pH balance. That's a normal process, but when those calcium reserves are called on too much, the bones will lose density and become brittle.

Hormone Imbalance

Yeasts, growing rapidly in the acidic environment they love, ferment hormones, decreasing the levels of DHEA, for one, and creating rampant imbalance among all hormones, resulting in such symptoms as hot flashes, bloating, water retention, irritability, and depression.

Sweating

You may find yourself breaking into a sweat while eating—officially, that's called gustatory sweating—while your body tries to get rid of the acid you're taking in via the pores of the skin.

Joint Problems

One disturbing hallmark of diabetes is called Charcot's joints. It most often affects weight-bearing joints such as the ankles. Bones weaken (as calcium is pulled out to neutralize acid), on top of which sensation is diminished (especially in the extremities) due to nerve damage, and so bone fractures can occur and yet go unnoticed, despite swelling. Because little pain is detected through those damaged nerves, the joint keeps getting used, the injury worsens, muscles shrink, and the joint can become permanently deformed.

Less initially dramatic, perhaps, but also common is finger stiffness, which can be severe enough to make it difficult to write, dress, tie shoes, or pick up small objects.

Periodontal Disease

Aggressive periodontal disease, gum-line cavities, dry mouth, and infections in the mouth are common in people with insulin resistance and Type 2 diabetes.

WATCH YOUR MOUTH

You can check the local acid level in your mouth with litmus paper; it should run between 6.8 and 7.2. Cutting out sugars and carbohydrates on the pH Miracle plan will protect your teeth as well. Brush your teeth after each meal with an alkaline toothpaste (any baking soda toothpaste; see the resources section) or a paste of distilled water and sodium bicarbonate (baking soda). Be sure to use a soft nylon brush with rounded ends on the bristle, and make sure to brush your tongue as well. Rinse your mouth with a solution of sodium silicate, sodium chlorite, or high pH (9.5 pH) water in the morning upon rising and at bedtime.

Yeast Infections

Vaginal yeast infections are just one obvious manifestation of yeast overgrowth in the body, and women with diabetes get them more often than women with normal blood sugar levels.

I'm quite sure there's nothing on this list you'd want to experience if you didn't have to. For years, these problems have been treated as all but inevitable in the wake of a diabetes diagnosis. So I can't say it loud or often enough: Maintaining consistently good blood sugar control can prevent these complications. Insulin and oral medications have side effects of their own, and their coverage can be spotty anyway, especially with the sugary diets they support. The pH Miracle plan controls blood sugar once and for all, naturally, and with no side effects. Or rather, with only *positive* side effects! With it, you can cross each and every one of the issues in this chapter off your list of things to worry about.

Chapter 4

The Cycle of Imbalance and Balance

Disease is born of us and in us.
—Antoine Bechamp

I believe the Law of Opposites is a major foundation of the universe, and that in many ways our mission is to find the balance between two poles. This book deals with one of the biggies: the imbalance that sickness and disease reveal, and the balance represented by health and fitness.

As in all of nature, the body tries to maintain a balance of influences in its own inner landscape or terrain. The most important of the many factors involved in this is the biochemical balance between acid and alkaline in the fluids of the blood and tissues. You don't need to grasp all the detailed biochemistry here; the take-home message is that acid and alkaline (or acid and base) are polar opposites, like hot and cold. When they meet in certain concentrations, they cancel each other out. In your body, it takes twenty parts alkaline to neutralize one part acid. The acid–alkaline relationship is measured as pH (after the "power of hydrogen").

Your body is pH-balanced at 7.365, and will do anything, even at the expense of your bones and other tissues, to keep the blood at that level. The acceptable pH level for urine and saliva ranges a bit more widely, from 6.8 to 7.2. That's my opinion; mainstream medical science is happy with a pH between 5.5 and 6.5. But those levels, while they may be "normal"—in that more people fall in that range than don't—are actually too acidic, a sign of too much sugar and other carbs in the diet. When the pH of the urine and/or saliva falls below 6.0, more than likely the pancreas and hormone-releasing adrenal glands will be stressed out and the body will be in a prediabetic state. (See chapter 2 for information on diagnosing diabetes the traditional way, via blood sugar levels.)

CYCLE OF IMBALANCE

Imagine not taking out the garbage around your house for a year. Besides the incredibly disgusting mess itself, you'd also have all kinds of critters taking up residence with you. A year of living and eating dangerously dirties your inner environment in the same way, and makes a warm welcome for microscopic critters that should give you the same shivers as the thought of rats or roaches in your house.

You have entered what I call the Cycle of Imbalance. It's the pathway to all sickness and disease, including hypo- and hyperglycemia and Type 1 and 2 diabetes, and it has four stages:

Stage 1: A physical or even emotional disturbance to the environment. In the case of diabetes, this might mean a megadose of sugar, or a diet generally high in sugars. It might also mean negative thoughts, words, or deeds; destructive emotions (as we'll see in chapter 6); or a polluted external environment (as with carbon monoxide from cars and trucks, or electromagnetic frequencies).

Stage 2: Disorganization of the cell and its microzymas. As the cell disorganizes, more acids are created, compromising the internal environment further still.

Stage 3: As the cells adapt to their increasingly acidic environment, they begin to change their form and function, becoming bacteria, then yeasts, then molds, and, eventually, microzymas.

Stage 4: These new biological forms ferment the body's glucose (leading to hypoglycemia, and so forth), then its fats, and, finally, its protein, creating still more debilitating acids—which start this vicious cycle all over again.

The symptoms we get—and cluster together and label as disease—are nothing more than the body's attempt to maintain its delicate pH balance and escape the Cycle of Imbalance. In the early stages of imbalance, symptoms may be relatively minor: headaches, skin eruptions, allergies, sinus problems, inflammation and irritation, and so on. These early signs are often treated with drugs, though all that really does is mask the problem, rather than eliminating it. In fact, major manipulation of symptoms contributes to *intensifying* those same symptoms down the line.

As things get farther out of whack, weakened organs and systems (the pancreas, for instance) start to give out in major ways. Fortunately, we know how to sidestep the cycle altogether—it's under your control. You don't "get" diabetes—you "do" it. If you do the things that get and keep you in the Cycle of Imbalance, threatening your body's pH balance and forcing it to flail about every which way to try to maintain it, you're "doing" diabetes. A number of things can put you into that cycle, the main ones being poor food choices and poor digestion, and you'll learn more about them in upcoming chapters.

CYCLE OF BALANCE

On the other hand, you can choose instead the Cycle of Balance, keeping your body in pH balance and maintaining stable, healthy blood sugar levels. It will help you reclaim your internal terrain and stop being poisoned by debilitating acids. This is the pathway to health, energy, and vitality.

The Cycle of Balance has three stages. They are easy to remember as "the 3Cs": cleanse, control, and construct:

Stage 1: Cleanse your body from the inside out, eliminating the acid wastes from being in imbalance, with plenty of water, green foods, and green drinks, as outlined in chapter 7.

Stage 2: Control your negative habits of eating, thinking, and living, breaking the pattern of disturbances in your body.

Stage 3: Construct new and healthy cells by providing your body with strong foundational materials, including water, oxygen, nutritious foods, vitamins, minerals, herbs, cell salts, and an overall lifestyle aimed at keeping your body alkaline. (More about all this in the following chapters.)

As you move through these stages, all your body systems will begin working together to bring harmony and balance, and you will notice the emergence of the signs of true good health: energy, mental clarity, clear and bright eyes, and a lean and trim body.

BETA CELL BURNOUT

We're not done with vicious cycles yet. As I've already mentioned, all diabetic symptoms, including obesity, skin problems, foot problems, gum disease, kidney disease, neuropathy, nerve damage, cardiovascular disease, hyper- or hypoinsulinemia, and hyper- or hypoglycemia, can be traced back through the eight steps of beta cell burnout, all of which reinforce each other and magnify the end results:

1. A diet high in sugar leads to
2. Hyperglycemia (high blood sugar), which signals
3. The release of insulin from the pancreas, and, if the above two continue, eventual hyperinsulinemia, which leads to
4. Pancreatic insufficiency, including breakdown of the beta cells and hypoinsulinemia, as well as reduced pancreatic enzymes and increased acidity in the small intestine, creating
5. Acidification of the body, leading to
6. Blood cells beginning to break down into bacteria and yeast, which have a ferocious appetite for sugar and rapidly ferment those sugars into acidic wastes, so the body gets more and more out of pH balance, reinforcing this whole cycle and setting the stage for

7. Insulin resistance and ever-more-compromised inner terrain, even higher blood sugar, insulin release, and acidity, ultimately creating
8. Diabetic symptoms.

ALPHA CELL BURNOUT

As the acid and yeast build up, blood sugar ferments, and hypoglycemia kicks in from runaway insulin release, the alpha cells as well as the beta cells get worn out and ineffective. My own research always shows biological transmutations of body cells to bacteria and yeast in the blood of people with hypoglycemia. In yet another vicious cycle, an array of secondary diabetic symptoms results, including yeast infections, muscle soreness, muscle wasting, being underweight, fatigue and tiredness, depression, dizziness, muddled thinking, and cardiovascular problems. There are six steps:

1. Blood sugar drops.
2. Alpha cells kick in, converting and releasing sugar into the blood.
3. Rising blood sugar and acid levels (from fermentation of sugar).
4. Hypoglycemia, and sugar building up in tissues.
5. Acidic tissue.
6. Diabetic symptoms.

The only way to break these cycles is to leave behind the whole Cycle of Imbalance, living by the principles outlined in following chapters to maintain the Cycle of Balance.

THE PANCREAS

The first line of defense when it comes to maintaining the critical alkaline environment in your body is your pancreas. The pancreas is a large gland, about the size of your fist and weighing about 8 ounces, located toward the back of the abdominal cavity, behind and below the stomach. Isolated clusters of cells known as the islets of Langerhans are scattered throughout the pancreas, and they are capable of measuring blood sugar levels every ten seconds, within a 2 percent range of accuracy. The islets give the pancreas its most famous role in diabetes, that of regulating the level of sugar in the blood: They are home to the beta and alpha cells responsible for producing insulin and glucagon, respectively. Insulin helps transport sugar in the blood into our seventy-five trillion cells, for energy. Glucagon signals the liver and the muscles when to convert their stored glycogen back into glucose (a process called glycogenolysis), to raise blood sugar.

But the pancreas has another, equally important role in diabetes (or lack thereof) as well. Because your stomach is, by design, an acidic environment, partially digested food is generally acidic as it moves out of the stomach, even on the healthiest diet. The pancreas secretes digestive enzymes into the small intestine to balance out the acidity and maintain an alkaline environment in the small intestine. In helping digest proteins, in particular, the pancreas is crucial to making sure the body has access to all the amino acids (the building blocks of protein) it needs to make insulin in the quantity—and of the quality—needed. Those amino acids are also necessary for making more digestive enzymes.

When our diet is continually full of acid-producing foods (more about which in chapter 7), it puts a lot of ongoing stress on the pancreas as it struggles to maintain the pH balance in the small intestine. The secretion of the alkalinizing enzyme is often inhibited in an overacidic body. As the pancreas itself becomes more acidic, it is less and less able to work to reduce acidity—or produce insulin. On all but a highly alkaline diet, any food and drink then simply creates more acidity, and without the pancreas kicking in its alkaline secretions, the organism (that's you!) is doomed to cellular breakdown and death.

Ken's Story

I've been a Type 1 diabetic for over thirty years—since I was five years old. I maintained generally excellent health for most of that time through my martial arts practice. But I stopped working out four years ago when my second child was born. My health has been deteriorating ever since.

I became depressed. I put on weight. I always felt exhausted. I was gulping down four 20-ounce cups of coffee and sometimes taking caffeine pills just to make it through the day. All this while I was taking an antidepressant that was supposedly improving my mood.

With all this going on, my A1c (a measure of blood sugar; see chapter 6) was 8.3 (diabetic range). I was tipping the scales at 212 pounds. Finally, my doctor said I *had* to get my diabetes under control. If I kept on going how I was, I was looking at an early and ugly death. He told me to lose some weight and exercise more. I was feeling so bad, I knew he was right. I had to do something.

So, Thanksgiving weekend I started drinking green drink with pH drops, and started changing to an alkaline diet. In three days, I was off coffee, without side effects. In three months, I lost over 30 pounds; I'm down to 182 pounds. I need 50 percent less insulin in the daytime, sometimes skipping insulin altogether while still maintaining low blood sugars. I've cut back my nighttime dose as well.

At a checkup, my doctor told me I looked great, and to keep doing whatever I was doing: My A1c was 7.0—nondiabetic. My blood sugars, which had consistently averaged over 200 as I tested them six times a day, were now staying in the 125 range, a normal, nondiabetic average. My energy is back up, and I am exercising again.

Staying with this program is not easy. People ask me how I can do it so consistently. But how could I not? It's given me what I've wished for for decades: hope of a cure of my diabetes. I'm thrilled just to be keeping it in check. For the first time in my life, this program has given me a bright future.

HOW OUR BODIES PRODUCE ENERGY

Food is a complex mixture of carbohydrates, fats, proteins, minerals, and other molecules that your body must convert into energy to keep itself running. Your digestive system, including the pancreas, handles the first step in the journey from food to energy. Digesting food is just a process of breaking down a diverse array of complex molecules into a small number of simpler ones. Proteins are broken down into amino acids. Fats are split into fatty acids and glycerol. And complex carbohydrates and sugars such as those found in fruits and grains are converted into simple sugars like glucose (the sugar with the simplest structure of all).

The cells of the body convert sugar into the energy they need to function. Your metabolic system then breaks apart those simple molecules to release their stored energy and capture it in molecules of ATP (adenosine triphosphate). The sugar is oxidized—processed with the addition of oxygen—into water, carbon dioxide, and ATP. The body requires oxygen to complete the conversion beneficially, the same way fire requires oxygen. Without oxygen, metabolism becomes a fermentation process, and the end result is lactic acid and carbonic acid rather than ATP energy. (This is an important point to remember when we get to chapter 9 on exercise, because overexercising creates a state of oxygen deprivation in the body. Eating a lot of sugar does the same.) Excess acid, of course, compromises the delicate pH balance of your body fluids.

While sugar is generally burned off as it is taken in, fat is mainly stored up. Some is in short-term storage, but most is not immediately called on and so is quickly squirreled away as reserves meant to last over the long haul. It takes a very short time to change food fat into body fat. There are vast storage depots all over the body, and there is fatty tissue in every organ (so that if it is ever called on, it can be conveniently delivered where it's needed). Not that any of this will come as much of a surprise to anyone who has looked around at Americans' bodies lately!

Stored fat can be burned to fuel the body's energy requirements, and body fat is in fact constantly being formed and broken down. But as long as sugar is available, the body will use that to power itself. Were you to stop eating—and so stop supplying sugar—the body would begin to live on its stored fat. This kind of fat-burning metabolism will give you about twice as much energy as sugar metabolism running on carbohydrates will. Burning fat for energy requires less energy. Plus, burning fat is a much cleaner source of fuel than carbs/sugars and creates less acidic pollution, less stress on the beta and alpha cells of the pancreas. Some of the breakdown products of dietary fat can be used to create ATP energy, but skipping the acid-producing part of the sugar-centered process. Still, your body won't use this pathway if there's sugar around to ease it down a different road.

Chapter 5

You Are Overacid,
Not Overweight

*Let us first understand the facts,
and then we may seek the cause.*
—ARISTOTLE

Americans have never been more overweight. New statistics reveal that a startling 64 percent of adults—120 million people—weigh too much. That's the highest rate ever recorded, and an increase of more than 60 percent just since 1991. Thirty-one percent of people over twenty are obese (30 or more pounds above healthy body weight calculated in relation to height, or more than 20 percent above ideal body weight); the remaining group, more than one in three Americans, are "only" overweight (10 to 30 pounds above healthy body weight). Five percent of adults are extremely obese, more than 50 pounds above healthy body weight, up from 3 percent just a decade ago. And researchers of one of the largest studies tracking down these statistics firmly believe that their numbers are actually an *under*estimate of the problem.

We are in the midst of an epidemic of obesity.

More women are obese than men (33 versus 28 percent). And black women as a group have the most dramatic statistic in this area: 50 percent of black women are obese (15 percent extremely obese), compared to 40 percent of Mexican American women and 30 percent of white women. (There is virtually no difference in rates of obesity among men based on race.) Rates are rising faster than average among thirty-somethings (up more than 70 percent over the course of the 1990s), and among people with at least some college education.

Worse still, these rates are surely going to increase further: 13 to 14 percent of American children and teenagers are already over-weight—that's nine million kids—with another seven million con-sidered "at risk" of joining that group. The rate of overweight children has risen rapidly over recent years—tripling, in fact, in the last two decades—and likely will continue to increase. Rates of obe-sity among teens have risen even faster than those among middle-aged adults. Children who are overweight are more likely to be overweight as adults, and incur the same increases in health risks.

Already obesity is rapidly catching up to tobacco as the top health threat in this country, according to the CDC's recent recalcu-lation of actual causes of death in the United States.

All this has ominous implications for the rates of heart disease and diabetes in the country—already so overwhelming—and a host of other devastating conditions directly affected by weight. Medical risks increase with weight, including the risk of developing diabetes and all the problems associated with it. Overweight children are at increased risk of a wide range of health problems, including Type 2 diabetes, which was almost unknown in children until about thirty years ago. More than half of the deaths of American women can be attributed to obesity. Excess weight is responsible for more than 325,000 premature deaths each year in this country, second only to tobacco-related deaths (430,000 killed each year). But smoking rates, at least, are going down. Yet obesity rates have tripled, and obesity is fast becoming the leading cause of death in America. And still Americans get fatter and fatter, apparently heedless of more than forty years of medical advice on losing weight by eating less and exercising more.

YOUR FAT MAY BE SAVING YOUR LIFE

It would seem that our fat is killing us. And far be it from me to argue for carrying around excess baggage. But the truth is, right now all that fat is probably *saving* your life. That's because the body uses fat to bind up and neutralize its excess acids, protecting all the tissues and organs that sustain life from acid damage. The bound acid can then be eliminated or—and here's the catch—stored. Storing acid in the fat keeps it away from the critical organs, but those fat depots create their own long-term health problems. Still, this helps explain why thin people are not necessarily healthier than fat people: The fat is providing a place to park acids, which in thin people may be free to break down body tissues, causing an array of symptoms. Next time you're jealous of those thin people we all know who can eat anything and everything without ever gaining an ounce, you might want to think twice: They are actually facing a serious problem because the fat buffering system of the body is not working properly.

Thus, overweight and underweight (which is common in Type 1) are two sides of the same coin. But in general, the more acidic your lifestyle and diet, the fatter you will be. Faced with all the sugars and acids deluging it every day, the body has only one choice to protect itself: fat. The corresponding good news is that the less acidic your lifestyle and diet, the thinner you will be, since your body won't need all that fat stored up just to save you from acidity. Your problems don't, at the root, come from being overweight—they come from being overacid.

There is a long list of fat's other beneficial roles in the body. First and foremost, fat is the body's best source for clean energy. (Upcoming chapters will show you how to eat right to get your body burning fat, rather than sugar, to power itself.) Fat stored under the skin insulates our bodies and helps keep us warm. The fat around joints and nerves, and between muscle fibers, protects against injury. Fat helps to hold some organs, like the kidneys, in their proper positions in the body. Fat is at the foundation of all hormone production.

All this goes to show: Fat is truly your friend. But it has to be the right kind of fat. And as with anything else, you want to avoid too much of a good thing.

YOUR CHOLESTEROL MAY BE
SAVING YOUR LIFE

We are almost as afraid of high cholesterol as we are of fat. But cholesterol is another binder of acids in the body. The body's self-preservation mode in the face of excess acidity involves creating those "bad cholesterol" LDLs (low-density lipoproteins) out of fat to help get rid of the acid. Excess LDL builds up in your arteries, contributing to heart disease. The bottom line here is going to sound familiar: Eliminate your acidic lifestyle and diet, and you will help lower your cholesterol.

(Cholesterol actually serves many important functions in the body, and cholesterol found in the skin, for example, can be converted into vitamin D when exposed to sunlight. Bile salts are derived from cholesterol. Cholesterol is involved in sex hormone and steroid hormone production by the adrenal gland, especially in times of severe stress. In short: Scientists have come to realize that cholesterol is necessary for the optimum health of the whole person—and that's before it has even come into being properly recognized for the acid defense that it is.)

THE RISKS OF OBESITY

This section might also be called "The Risks of Acidity." To my mind, it's pretty much one and the same thing. You shouldn't blame your fat for your health problems—without it, they'd be even worse. Losing weight may reduce some of your risks, but until you deal with the underlying problem—until you get rid of the acid—you won't find your way to true and lasting good health. Some of the major risks generally associated with obesity, which are also inextricably linked to acidity, include hyperglycemia, hypoglycemia, heart disease, arthritis, liver disease, kidney disease, bad skin, and, of course, diabetes.

Pat's Story

I have Type 2 diabetes, which I control by diet alone, thanks to green drinks with pH drops and eating alkaline food. My doctors recommended oral medications, but I keep my blood sugar levels under control on my own this way, and I've lowered my blood pressure as well. And, I lost 30 pounds. Not to mention the energy and feeling of well-being I get with the green drinks.

We've already looked at how hypo- and hyperglycemia and heart disease relate to acidity. They aren't the only ones, of course. Arthritis, for example, stems from the body's use of calcium to bind acids. The resulting microcalcifications build up in the joints, stiffening them and making movement painful. The liver is a major filter for toxins in the body, including acids, and it can handle only so much before it breaks down. When the liver can't manage the acids, the kidneys are your next line of defense, and they, too, eventually get overwhelmed and break down. When the liver and kidneys can't keep up with filtering out the acid in our bodies, acid comes right out through our "third kidney"—the skin—leading to acne, blemishes, rash, eczema, psoriasis, and more.

KETONES AND KETOACIDOSIS

For people with Type 1 diabetes, one severe complication always has to be of concern: ketoacidosis, or very high blood glucose with large amounts of ketones in the blood. Ketones are acids produced from fat metabolism (ketosis) when your body doesn't have enough insulin and is already overacidic. But when you are eating right, ketosis is actually a good thing.

Without insulin, or without enough chromium to bind insulin to sugar, sugar can't get into the cells. Thus your body cannot fuel itself with sugar, and an alternative source of energy is needed. So it begins to burn fat instead—it goes into ketosis. This is the good news, since fat metabolism is the healthiest way to create energy, producing twice the amount of energy as sugar metabolism or protein metabolism with half the amount of waste. If you're eating to keep your body pH-balanced, the small amount of waste created will be quickly and easily eliminated from your body. If your body is acidic, however, the resulting ketones are not eliminated (via cholesterol, calcium, or other buffers), and they can build up in your blood, compromising your body's delicate pH balance and causing it to go into ketoacidosis. And that's *not* good. The body goes into preservation mode, using body fluids to dilute and neutralize the acid, leading to nausea, vomiting, dehydration, rapid breathing, and muscle soreness. If you don't deal with ketoacidosis appropriately, it can lead to diabetic coma, and eventually kill you.

In ketoacidosis, blood sugars are usually above 300 mg/dl, or 16.6 mmol/liter, and urine will be 2 percent sugar or more. You can get products that test your urine for ketones—including Acetest tablets, Ketostix, and Chemstrip K—at a pharmacy, without a prescription. There is also an instrument sold as Precision Xtra, which tests ketones in the blood. Test your ketones in the morning or at night before going to bed, following the instructions that come with the product you choose, and be sure your timing is accurate. If there is no color change in the ketone strip, you are not burning ketones/ fat but are still relying on burning sugar for energy. You'll need to include more good fats in your diet to help your body move away from the sugar. If the strip begins to change color by moving toward beige or brown, then you are burning fat rather than sugar.

If tests show ketones in your urine, and your blood sugar is above 300 mg/dl or has risen over the past twelve hours, and/or you have nausea or vomiting, call your doctor, begin superhydrating the body with alkalizing fluids (see chapter 7), and measure your sugar and ketone levels again after half an hour.

Over the long term, you can help prevent ketoacidosis by eating right, of course, and also by taking chromium and vanadium to help bind insulin to glucose, and by supporting the pancreas and adrenals with nutritional supplements (see chapter 8).

Erica's Story

I'd been gaining weight continually and inexplicably for years until I was finally diagnosed as insulin-resistant. I began taking a green drink with pH drops and noticed a marked improvement in my energy level; I even lost a few pounds. I also noticed I didn't have my usual PMS or ragweed allergies. Realizing I could do even better, I began adding fresh raw vegetables to my diet in large quantities. Before I knew it, the weight was falling off and my blood sugar had dropped 15 points. Now I was really motivated, and decided to do even more, so I went on a four-day liquid feast. I felt so much better afterward (realized I didn't need anti-inflammatories after a long day at my desk anymore), and lost even more weight. Seven weeks into the program, I am down 12 pounds and, more importantly, my blood sugar is 80! What's more, I've been able to stop (with my doctor's supervision) taking the antidepressants I've been on for the last five years. I am officially no longer insulin-resistant, and I couldn't be more thrilled.

FAT AND DIABETES

Even if we have yet to determine the causal link, what's clear is that obesity and diabetes go hand in hand. A huge study published in the *Journal of the American Medical Association* tracking the increasing rate of obesity in this country—finding a jump of more than 5 percent just from 2000 to 2001—also found an increase over the same period of more than 8 percent in the rate of diabetes. (Other health conditions linked to being overweight—including cardiovascular disease, stroke, and cancer, to name just a few—are also on the rise, no surprise. Excess weight causes at least three hundred thousand deaths each year, not to mention in excess of $117 billion in health care costs.)

We can see the overweight–diabetes association clearly in children as well. As childhood obesity has grown more and more common, doctors have noted the increasing incidence of Type 2 diabetes— which not long ago had an average age of onset of *sixty*. More than three hundred thousand American children now have Type 2 diabetes, with all its attendant risk of serious complications, including blindness, kidney failure, and stroke. A quarter of obese children younger than ten, and a fifth of obese adolescents, have impaired glucose tolerance, the first step on the road to diabetes. Clearly, the condition is called Type 2 because the term *adult-onset diabetes* no longer applies.

In 2001, the *New England Journal of Medicine* published a study that followed more than eighty-four thousand women over sixteen years, tracking their weight, diet, exercise, smoking, and alcohol consumption. Over the course of the study, thirty-three hundred women developed Type 2 diabetes—and being overweight was the single most important predictor of which of the women they would be, followed by lack of exercise, poor diet, and current smoking. The full results of the study suggested that more than 90 percent of cases of Type 2 diabetes could be prevented if everyone adopted a healthy lifestyle that included a good diet (see chapter 7), regular exercise (see chapter 9), maintaining an appropriate weight, and avoiding cigarettes.

Eighty percent of diabetics are too fat. All are too acidic. Ironically, what they need is often *more* fat—but of the right kind and in the right places. How to ensure that is the lesson in chapter 7: adding good fats to the diet, eliminating excessive sugars, teaching the body to burn fat rather than sugar. Revamping your metabolism this way allows the body to heal the pancreas, eventually leading to the reversal and even cure of diabetes. Now the choice is yours: Will fat kill you, or save your life?

Chapter 6

The pH Miracle for
Type 1 and Type 2 Diabetes

Man can learn nothing unless he proceeds
from the known to the unknown.
—CLAUDE BERNARD

Reversing hyperglycemia, hypoglycemia, and Type 1 and 2 diabetes is as straightforward as maintaining a pH balance in your body. If you significantly reduce the acid your body receives and makes due to your diet and lifestyle, you'll provide the proper alkaline environment your body needs for true good health.

Let this chapter be your official invitation to change your body—and your life—forever with the pH Miracle plan. This is *not* a treatment, but a way of living, a way of eating, even a way of thinking. If you want to truly be free of your diabetes, you will have to change. The change in many cases is drastic. Only you can say if it is worth it. But I dare you: Put a price on life, and on a life full of true energy and fitness, and joy, peace, harmony, and love. You could have all the money in the world, but without your health you'd have *nothing*.

This chapter outlines the basic steps of the pH Miracle plan, though diet, supplements, and exercise will be discussed in more detail in following chapters. As you read the 10 Steps to a Cure here, keep in mind what Jesus said about all things being possible for those who believe. Have faith in knowing that the only constant in life is change. When you change the environment, everything within that new environment will change. Like placing a snowball on your kitchen counter and watching it transform totally with the change of environment, following these steps will allow you to witness the profound change in yourself as you change your body's inner environment.

10 STEPS TO A CURE—THE pH MIRACLE LIFESTYLE AND DIET

No less a mainstream authority than the *New England Journal of Medicine* declared that nine out of ten cases of Type 2 diabetes could be prevented if people exercised more, ate better, stopped smoking, and adopted other healthy behaviors. I've set my sights for you even higher. With the pH Miracle plan, preventing, or even reversing, diabetes—even Type 1 diabetes—is the goal.

The basic components are hydration (lots of alkaline water), eating alkaline foods, supplementation, and exercising (properly). The full program breaks down into ten steps. I'm going to set out all the steps for you here very briefly, so you can get the lay of the land. I'll go into more detail in the rest of the chapter, with some steps then developed into chapters of their own:

1. See your doctor for a thorough physical.
2. Check your sugar levels daily.
3. Go on a fourteen-day liquid feast.
4. Eat an alkaline diet.
5. Begin a program of nutritional supplements.
6. Drink your greens.
7. Exercise (appropriately) every day.
8. Manage your stress levels.
9. Monitor your progress.
10. Pursue a positive attitude.

Arthur's Story

I was diagnosed with Type 1 diabetes just after I turned nine years old, so I've had more than twenty years' experience in dealing with it. Nothing prepared me for what incredible results I would get with the pH Miracle, or the short amount of time it took to achieve them.

I saw a dramatic drop in my insulin needs and blood sugar levels as I was starting the program with the liquid feast. As I came off it, I was still gradually reducing my dosages following my body's decreasing need for the artificial insulin. I am now using more than 80 percent less insulin than I started on.

That's not all. I'm especially gratified by the evidence that I'm beating all the side effects of out-of-control blood sugar and insulin levels, as well as beating the diabetes. I've lost not only my much-hated "love handles," but also the 50 pounds that accompanied them. My tastes have changed, and I can't believe how delicious all the wonderful vegetables and spices are. Plus, I no longer have those devastating carbohydrate cravings. My cholesterol level has improved. My vision has improved.

What's more, now I find it easy to get out of bed in the morning, and I have plenty of energy throughout the day. My allergies and constant nasal infections are gone. I keep expecting the cold sores I've had sporadically since I was a teenager to show back up, but they don't. I no longer catch every cold that's going around.

For me, it truly has been a pH miracle.

STEP 1: LET'S GET (A) PHYSICAL

Your first stop should be your doctor's office for a thorough medical history and physical exam. The American Diabetes Association recommends that all adults over forty-five be tested for diabetes, though

I'd encourage everyone to get tested, especially if you have any other symptoms. The key test is a check of your fasting blood glucose levels—that is, a laboratory check of your blood following a fast of at least eight hours. A reading of 110 mg/dl or under is considered normal, and if you fall here the ADA guidelines state that you should simply be retested every three years. If your results are between 110 and 125 mg/dl, consider yourself at high risk of diabetes. More than 126 mg/dl, and you've bought yourself an official diabetes diagnosis.

Anyone having any prediabetic symptoms should also have a glucose tolerance test. First you'll have your blood drawn after fasting for at least eight hours to establish a baseline reading. You'll then take a sugar-water solution (I recommend one you make yourself, combining 12 ounces distilled water, 40 g sugar, and 1 g potassium) and thirty minutes later have your blood tested again, with additional readings forty-five minutes later, and twenty minutes after that. (See below for how to interpret the resulting curves.)

Diabetes doesn't affect only your blood sugar—effects are felt all over the entire body. Everyone should keep tabs on their overall health, and this is particularly important when there is a specific challenge to it, like diabetes. So a general, thorough physical is in order. It should include a check of blood pressure, pulse rate, breathing rate, temperature, eyes, ears, nose, and throat (including the thyroid gland). You should be interested in the results of several lab tests as well:

- *A complete blood count (CBC)* measures the number of various types of cells found in your blood, particularly red and white blood cells. A high level of white blood cells indicates a high level of biological transmutations, such as yeast and bacteria and their associated waste products (acids). A low level of red blood cells indicates a diet high in acidic food and too low in alkalinizing food, especially green foods and drinks, and resulting overacidity of the 9 yards' worth of intestines, especially the intestinal villis where the red blood cells are formed.
- *A standard blood chemistry profile* includes a battery of twelve to twenty-five chemical indicators of health, such as liver

enzymes, blood urea nitrogen (BUN), creatinine, alkaline phosphatase, calcium, and sodium. Potassium is crucial for keeping blood pH at the appropriate 7.365 level, so your doctor will want to check you have sufficient amounts: 4.5 to 5.5 mEq/liter. Magnesium reduces acidity and maintains body temperature. Low levels of red blood cell magnesium indicates a lack of green foods in the diet. Your triglycerides level will tell you your magnesium status. Normal triglycerides are between 90 and 110 mg/dl; high levels mean low magnesium. Low alkaline phosphatase levels also indicate magnesium deficiency. Normal values for men are 90 to 239 u/liter; for women under age forty-five, between 76 and 196 u/liter; and for women forty-five and older, between 87 and 250 u/liter. Children normally have levels three times those of adults.

- *A lipid profile* measures fatty substances—lipids—in the blood, including HDL and LDL cholesterol and total cholesterol, and triglycerides. High LDL indicates an overly acidic system.
- *A serum C-peptide test* measures C-peptide, a protein produced by the beta cells of the pancreas whenever insulin is made. The level of C-peptide in the blood, then, is an index of the amount of insulin you are producing. Type 1 diabetics have a level of 0, and those with mild Type 2, or insulin resistance, are usually within or above the "normal" range. High levels mean the beta cells are overreacting to increases in blood sugar.
- *A homocysteine test* measures an amino acid (homocysteine) that tends to be high in people with diabetes, as well as in people whose bodies are too acidic.
- *A thrombotic risk profile* measures whether you have a tendency to produce blood clots inappropriately, which can happen with high acidity due to high blood sugar. That's the acids, doing their thing as a kind of molecular glue, causing cells to stick together—even when it interferes with proper blood circulation.
- *A renal risk profile* via angiography or CT of the kidney rates your risk of kidney disease or dysfunction, another possible side effect of years of overacidity in the body.
- *A urine and saliva pH test, and a blood pH test,* can alert you if you are outside the normal ranges (6.8 to 7.2, and 7.365,

respectively). High blood pH indicates acid in the tissues as the body tries to maintain pH balance by throwing excess acids out into the tissues for the lymphatic system to deal with. Low blood pH indicates, of course, acids in the blood.

SAMPLE URINE pH CURVES			
	Ideal	Prediabetic	Severely Diabetic
Fasting	6.8–7.2	6.5	5.8
30 minutec after eating	5.6–5.8	5.8	5.6
+ 45 minutes	6.0–6.4	6.0	5.5
+ 20 minutes	6.6–6.8	6.2	5.3–5.4

- *A hemoglobin A1c test (or HgbA1c, HbA1c, or glycohemoglobin test)* measures the amount of glucose (sugar) that sticks to red blood cells. It gives you an estimated average of hemoglobin molecules that contain sugar over the life of a red blood cell (120 days). Think of it as an average of all your blood sugars for that period of time. The normal value is generally about 4 to 6 percent, so ask your doctor for the range you should fall into. Usually, up to 7 percent is considered acceptable, with 8 percent or higher marking a diabetes diagnosis. People with diabetes should have a hemoglobin A1c done every three months. Everyone should have it done at least as a baseline measurement.

Those with diabetes should also get regular neurological exams, checking for sensation in the feet and toes, reflexes of limbs and eyes, short-term memory, and muscle strength. They should also have a thorough eye exam every one to two years, frequent dental checkups, and regular foot examinations by a podiatrist.

HEALING FOOT ULCERS

Foot ulcers resulting from poor circulation and nerve damage are a common side effect of diabetes. Following the pH Miracle plan will heal and/or prevent them. If you currently have ulcers, try soaking your feet in an alkaline bath of sodium bicarbonate (baking soda) or sodium chlorite.

STEP 2: WATCH YOUR BLOOD SUGAR

If you have diabetes, you need to monitor your blood sugar levels daily—but not only for the usual reasons your doctor will give you. Watching your levels closely when you follow the pH Miracle plan will let you see your blood sugar levels drop significantly—which impacts the amount of insulin you need. Don't be surprised if your need for insulin drops more than 50 percent in the first seventy-two hours on a low-carbohydrate, low-protein, high-*good*-fat diet such as the pH Miracle. People with Type 2 or gestational diabetes benefit from regular blood sugar testing, too.

The American Diabetes Association guidelines for interpreting blood sugar results are as follows:

ADA BLOOD SUGAR GUIDELINES			
	Fasting	*1¼–2 Hours After Eating*	*Bedtime*
Normal	Less than 110 mg/dl	Less than 140 mg/dl	Less than 120 mg/dl
Acceptable	80–120 mg/dl	Less than 80 mg/dl	100–140 mg/dl
Needs improvement	Under 80 mg/dl; over 140 mg/dl	More than 200 mg/dl	Under 100 mg/dl; over 160 mg/dl

Test your blood before all meals, one to two hours after meals, before you go to bed, and, if you are a Type 1 diabetic, at 2 or 3 A.M. Ideally, your blood sugar levels would look something like this: 80 mg/dl while you are fasting; thirty minutes after eating, 130; forty-five minutes later, 110; and 100 another twenty minutes after that, returning quickly thereafter to 80. You can see how that compares to diabetic and prediabetic results in the following chart:

SAMPLE BLOOD SUGAR RESULTS			
	Ideal	*Prediabetic*	*Severely Diabetic*
Fasting	80	80	140
30 minutes after eating	130	205	275
+ 45 minutes	110	200	285
+ 20 minutes	100	190	300

You may want to do tests more frequently when you are ill, if you suspect low blood sugar, before driving if you are taking insulin or sulfonylureas to lower blood sugar, when you are physically active, if you have frequent insulin reactions overnight, if you wake up with very high blood sugar, when you are changing your insulin injection plan, when you gain or lose weight, when you think you are pregnant or are considering getting pregnant, when your blood sugar levels have been dangerously low and high, and/or when you are on intensive insulin therapy.

The two methods available to you to test your blood sugar are the glucose meter and visual glucose strips. Glucose meters are battery-operated machines ranging from pen-sized to calculator-sized, weighing a few ounces. You place a drop of blood on a paper strip and insert the strip into the device, which then displays a numerical reading. Visual glucose strips are thin plastic strips with two small color blocks on them. When you put a drop of blood on the color blocks, they change color depending on the amount of sugar in the blood. You can identify your range by comparing the color to a color chart. You don't get an exact number this way, but rather a reading such as "low," "acceptable," or "too high." Any glucose meter or visual strip will provide you with an accurate blood sugar reading, assuming you follow the instructions carefully.

STEP 3: LIQUID FEAST

To make the most dramatic change in your life and health, and to get the most benefit out of the pH Miracle eating plan, you should begin with a fourteen- to twenty-one-day "liquid feast." Think of it as a bit of spring cleaning. The idea of the liquid feast, or cleanse, is to rid your body of the excess acid buildup from years of poor nutrition and high-sugar foods, get rid of negative microforms and their toxic wastes, detoxify your blood and tissues, normalize your blood sugar, and begin the process of healing your pancreas. It will also normalize digestion and metabolism, helping you regain pH balance.

Another reason we call this a cleanse will become quite apparent as you are going through it: This regimen will have a laxative effect on your system (which is exactly what you want). The acid wastes that are in your body won't just vanish, *poof!*—your body has to expel them. Until you see how your own body reacts to the liquid feast, plan to stay close to a bathroom—most people will need six to ten visits a day.

The exact length of the liquid feast phase will vary from person to person, depending on what your body needs and how your body reacts to it. Typically two weeks will give you the start you need to reverse your diabetes, though three is optimum.

Please note, this is not a fast! You will actually eat as much and as often as you want. Please eat until you are satisfied, not too full. The idea is to eat mainly green food (veggies), and to have them, for this opening phase, in a liquid form—pureed soups, or shakes, or juices. You'll have a few nongreen items as well: tomato, lemon, lime, bell pepper, jicama, and healthy oils.

Should you feel hunger pangs, remember that the first ones are usually the worst; eventually they will stop, and you may actually experience an upsurge in energy from all the alkaline food and drinks.

You should drink at least 4 liters of green drink a day, including (or in addition to) a liter of pure water and four 8-ounce glasses of fresh green vegetable juice (diluted with ten times as much water as juice). Try juicing cucumber, kale, broccoli, celery, lettuce, collards, okra, wheatgrass, barley grass, watercress, parsley, cabbage, spinach, and alfalfa sprouts. If you have low blood sugar, you can add a little carrot or beet juice, but remember that those vegetables are high in sugar, which juicing concentrates, so use them only as needed—and definitely avoid them if you are having hyperglycemia.

That's the "feast." The "liquid" part is there because everything you eat in this first phase should be pureed or juiced. That way, the food requires very little energy to digest. Normally, you use more than half your daily energy digesting. Removing that energy drain for a while means your body can use the bulk of its energy for regeneration of all your seventy-five trillion cells. Pureeing or juicing also makes the nutrients in food up to twenty times more available. Your body gets more water as well.

What follows is a schedule of a typical day on the liquid feast, plus a menu plan to guide you through these first two or three weeks. You'll find much more detail on food and water in chapter 7, and on supplements in chapter 8; and chapter 10 provides the recipes you'll need. But in general, here's a typical day:

7 A.M. (or, upon waking)
    1–1½ liters green drink or green shake (see page 107)
    Supplements
8 A.M.
    Soup
    Supplements
9 A.M.
    Supplements
9 A.M.–noon
    1–1½ liters green drink
10 A.M.
    Supplements
11:00 A.M.
    Supplements

1 P.M.

    Soup

    Supplements

2–5 P.M.

    1–1½ liters green drink

    Supplements

6 P.M.

    Soup

    Supplements

7–9 P.M.

    1–1½ liters green drink, or plain distilled water with sodium chlorite and lemon

    Supplements

You can adjust this as needed to fit your own daily schedule. Be sure to take capsule supplements with meals, and liquid supplements before meals. All soups should be pureed in a blender or food processor. If at any time during the day you are hungry, you can always have more soup or green drink. You can also juice fresh vegetables (no carrots or beets during this phase, because of their high sugar content, unless you are experiencing low blood sugar). See the Drinks and Shakes section in chapter 10 for recipes. You can maximize the alkalinizing effect of green vegetable juice by diluting it, one part juice to ten parts distilled water, and adding five drops of sodium chlorite or sodium silicate. As you'll see when you get to chapter 9, you should also plan on some time each day for exercising.

Each day follows the same basic outline as above, with a rotating cast of soups and shakes in the morning, midday, and evening, as follows:

Day 1

    Creamy Broccoli Soup (page 207)

    Popeye Soup (page 200)

    Healing Soup (page 203)

Day 2

    AvoRado Kid Super Green Shake (page 177)

    Madrid Gazpacho (from *pH Miracle*)

    AsparaZincado Soup (page 202)

Day 3

Celery Soup (page 204)

Madrid Gazpacho (from *pH Miracle*)

AsparaZincado Soup (page 202)

Day 4

Creamy Vegetable Soup (page 205; during the liquid feast, use 1½ cups fresh almond milk instead of tofu)

Mock Split Pea Soup (from *pH Miracle*)

Vegetable Minestrone Soup (from *pH Miracle*)

Day 5

Celery/Cauliflower Soup (page 206)

Chunky Veggie Soup (from *pH Miracle*)

Broccoli Creamed Soup (from *pH Miracle*)

Day 6

Popeye Soup (page 200)

Healing Soup (page 203)

AvoRado Kid Super Green Shake (page 177)

Day 7

Creamy Broccoli Soup (page 207)

Vegetable Minestrone Soup (from *pH Miracle*)

Green Power Cocktail (from *pH Miracle;* during the liquid feast, substitute celery or cucumber for the beets)

Day 8

Broccoli/Cauliflower Soup (page 205)

Madrid Gazpacho (from *pH Miracle*)

AvoRado Kid Super Green Shake (page 177)

Day 9

Green Raw Soup (page 202)

Creamy Broccoli Soup (page 207)

Healing Soup (page 203)

Day 10

Popeye Soup (page 200)

Celery/Cauliflower Soup (page 206)

Creamy Vegetable Soup (page 205; during the liquid feast, omit tofu, or use fresh almond milk instead)

Days 11–21

Repeat cycle, starting at Day 1.

Again, you can personalize this to your tastes as necessary. There's nothing magic about which dish you have at which meal, so if you want to pick a favorite to have every morning, or skip one you don't care for, or use up the veggies you have on hand, go right ahead.

STEP 4: AN ALKALINE DIET

Chapter 7 covers this subject in depth, so for now I just want to recommend an eating plan that is low in carbohydrates and protein and high in good fats. The specifics on the foods you should eat freely and what you should avoid are spelled out in the next chapter. As in the liquid feast, as long as you stick within the parameters of alkaline foods, you'll eat as much and as often as you want. You should never go hungry. But eat small meals many times a day (at least six, actually) rather than three large meals a day. Less more often is better than more less often.

The pH Miracle is really a lifetime plan—more a lifestyle than just a diet. You can't just conquer your diabetes by following the advice in this book, then go right back to eating and living the way you were before—unless you want your diabetes to come back. But once you experience how great you'll feel with a truly healthy body, I don't think you'll want to go back anyway.

This is meant to change your whole life, and the pH Miracle plan will eventually become something you do naturally, without having to think about it. Still, you should start out with a more structured approach. That's the official pH Miracle diet, a twelve- to sixteen-week program. It takes those three to four months to teach your cells a new way of living. Not to mention, *you* have to learn a new way of eating, thinking, and living. Neither one happens overnight. This is a process, not a onetime event.

STEP 5: SUPPLEMENTS

Chapter 8 lays out everything you need to know about using nutritional supplements—vitamins, minerals, cell salts, and herbs—with the pH Miracle plan for reversing diabetes. Using supplements correctly will support you through the change process, helping you cleanse your body and construct new and healthy cells. Supplements will help neutralize, bind, and eliminate acids, and turn bacteria and yeast back to helpful microzymas, bringing your body, naturally, back to a state of harmony and inner balance.

STEP 6: IT IS EASY, DRINKING GREEN

The next chapter also looks more closely at the importance of keeping your body hydrated with plenty of water—the right kind of water—and "green drink." Most people need at least 4 liters of green drink every day. I recommend 1 liter per day for every 30 pounds of body weight. This is critically important, because it lets the body move out acidic wastes and make its inner environment more alkaline, for healing and regeneration.

GREEN DRINK

Combine 1 liter or quart of distilled water with 16 drops sodium chlorite or sodium silicate and 1 teaspoon green powder. You can add 1 teaspoon of powdered soy sprouts, though that's optional. (Or, eat 1 teaspoon of soy sprout powder and then immediately drink your green drink.) Add some fresh lemon juice, if desired.

> ## Henry's Story
>
> I have had Type 2 diabetes since 1997. I was taking 2.5 mg of Glucotrol XL (an oral medication) and taking daily walks to control my blood sugars, but they were still too high. Until I started using a green drink with pH drops. I began keeping a chart to track my levels so I could see if I could detect any difference. Within two days, my readings were well within acceptable levels, and they've stayed there ever since, even when I stopped taking the Glucotrol. My diabetes is under control, and it appears the function of my pancreas has been restored. That is quite a miracle!

STEP 7: EXERCISE

You need daily exercise to keep your cells healthy and your body alkaline—yet exercise can acidify the body. The secrets to exercising right are explored in chapter 9. The good news is it takes just fifteen minutes a day to work the whole body in ways that increase blood circulation, decrease blood sugar, move acids out of the body, and make you stronger, more flexible, and, bottom line, healthier.

STEP 8: MANAGE YOUR STRESS LEVELS

Your emotions—good, bad, or indifferent—have a major impact on your pH balance and blood sugar levels. Your psychology affects your physiology—and your physiology affects your psychology.

Under stress, including the stress of powerful negative emotions such as anger, sadness, and fear, the adrenal glands release the fight-or-flight hormone adrenaline to help sustain your energy levels. Adrenaline signals the body to raise blood sugar levels, which signals the pancreas to release more insulin to bind to that sugar to take it into the cells for energy. All that is good, designed to provide a burst of energy to get you out of tight spots and over rough patches.

If that stress continues unrelievedly, however, you'll exhaust your adrenals and have no more resources to call on when the going gets tough. Your body cells will break down for sugar to keep up with the energy demands, and as a result your body gets more acidic as you enter the loop of insulin resistance and hypo- and hyperglycemia, probably with one or more of the telltale symptoms (light-headedness, dizziness, aches and pains, headache, upset stomach), and, ultimately, diabetes.

We all have stress in our daily lives, to a greater or lesser degree, and many times managing it is easier said than done. I recommend *Practicing the Power of Now* by Eckhart Tolle for those who would like help in learning how to manage stress.

To give you just one example of how mood connects to diabetes, consider a recent Japanese study demonstrating that diabetics better processed the sugar they consumed during meals if they ate while in a happy mood. Participants who ate while watching a comedy show had lower blood sugar levels afterward than did those who sat through a boring lecture—which held true for both those with Type 2 diabetes and those without diabetes. The researchers theorized that laughter might reduce blood sugar because it increases energy consumption, or because laughter affects the neuroendocrine system that controls blood sugar levels.

STEP 9: MONITOR YOUR PROGRESS

It can be hard to see how far you've come if you lose track of your starting point, not to mention the details of the journey. Keeping good records is very important to your quest to reverse diabetes. I recommend keeping a daily journal.

First of all, write down all your blood sugar readings, so you can see any patterns—and watch them stabilize thanks to your efforts. You'll find constant motivation to stick with this program there. Also, log in what you eat and drink, as well as all the nutritional supplements you

Daily Log

Date:_____ Weight (weekly): _____ A.M. Blood Sugar: _____ P.M. Blood Sugar: _____

Medication:

Name	Dosage	Time	
_____	_____	_____	A.M./P.M.
_____	_____	_____	A.M./P.M.
_____	_____	_____	A.M./P.M.
_____	_____	_____	A.M./P.M.
_____	_____	_____	A.M./P.M.
_____	_____	_____	A.M./P.M.
_____	_____	_____	A.M./P.M.
_____	_____	_____	A.M./P.M.
_____	_____	_____	A.M./P.M.
_____	_____	_____	A.M./P.M.

Supplements: (indicate times)

Green drink
pH drops
Soy sprouts
 powder
EFAs
Multi
Chromium/
 vanadium
NADP
Magnesium
Zinc
Herbal cleanser
Pancreas support
Other:

_____

_____

_____

_____

Food:
 Breakfast:
 Lunch:
 Dinner:
 Snacks:
 Water/juice:

Exercise:
 Type:
 Duration:

Notes:

take, so you can share this information with your doctor and see how it correlates with your blood sugar levels.

In addition, if you decide to write in a journal as one approach to managing stress (see above), you might want to incorporate that here as well. You may be surprised to find you can trace your moods and stress in relationship to your blood sugar levels.

Among other things, good records will let you see how well and quickly all the efforts you are making pay off. Many of my clients have needed to decrease the amount of insulin they take as much as 50 percent within just the first seventy-two hours.

STEP 10: THE POWER OF POSITIVE THINKING

Your success at curing your diabetes will depend in large part on your ability to pursue a positive attitude. Thoughts and emotions are very powerful, and only you can control them. Positive thoughts and emotions help maintain harmony and homeostasis within you, physically as well as psychically, while negative ones foster the breakdown of cells, the release of sugars, and the buildup of excess acidity.

The best way to stay emotionally balanced (and physically alkaline) is to focus on the present, on the moment you are living, on what is happening right now. Try not to live in the past or the future, and enjoy and treasure the here and now. Good thoughts, good words, and good deeds energize and alkalinize your body.

In addition, you may need your positive attitude to keep you on track with this plan, at least in the beginning. Change is never easy, and you'll be doing a major overhaul here. The beginning of the liquid feast in particular can be difficult as your body rids itself of so much accumulated toxic waste. But I think you'll find that the plan will soon start providing you with positive thinking, as you'll feel your success deep within you. It happens on such a profound level, and in such an overarching manner, that it tells you all you'll ever need to know about the rightness of this path for you. Soon enough, you won't need to consciously try to be positive about it—its positive nature will be manifest for all to see, and you'll naturally feel positive as a result.

Chapter 7

Let Food Be Your Medicine . . .

Let food be your medicine, and medicine your food.
—HIPPOCRATES

There's nothing complicated about eating to stabilize your blood sugar. Eat plenty of less acidic food, and skip the very acidic foods. You need to eat lots of green vegetables, (good) water, and (good) fats. You need to *not* eat sugars and starches. You need to eat frequently, and you need to *stop* eating when you are satisfied.

That's it. Follow these guidelines, and all your cells will be able to get and use all the energy they need without getting overwhelmed by sugar. Diabetes and the host of health problems that come with it will be a thing of the past. You'll need to support your body with nutritional supplements and appropriate exercise, but the centerpiece of the pH Miracle plan is your food. Just remember, when you fill up your tank, you deserve Premium. Don't bother with the junk; stick with nature's wholesome bounty for glowing good health.

A decade-long National Institutes of Health (NIH) study of Type 1 diabetes found that those who kept their blood sugar levels near normal cut their risk of eye, kidney, and nerve damage up to 70 percent. Uncontrolled sugar levels, however, increased the risk of blindness, heart disease, stroke, kidney failure, nerve damage, skin problems, and more. The landmark 2001 NIH clinical trial Diabetes Prevention Program showed conclusively that diet and exercise slash the risk of Type 2 diabetes by up to 58 percent.

And that's with a very conventional diet approach. My own fif-teen years of experience, research, and two recent controlled studies show that the pH Miracle plan does much, much better. And it helps prevent, improve, or reverse not only Type 2 diabetes, but Type 1 as well. Furthermore, the type and quality of fuel you put into your body determines whether or not you "graduate" from hypo- or hyper-glycemia to diabetes. An acidic diet will eventually push the body right over the borderline, while an alkaline diet will help prevent you from ever hearing that diagnosis.

All that thanks mainly to greens and good fats.

FAT METABOLISM

The underlying idea here is to teach your body to burn fat for energy rather than sugar or protein. On the standard American diet (SAD, indeed), you're running mainly on sugar. But fat is a much cleaner fuel, and it doesn't leave behind the toxic wastes sugar metabolism does. Using fat metabolism also gives your pancreas a break, and allows the body to begin healing the pancreas and its insulin-producing beta cells. Revolutionizing the way you eat can help prevent and reverse diabetes (as well as heart disease and the other negative side effects of diabetes).

LESS IS MORE

It's not only *what* you eat, but also *how* you eat that's important for good health. You must eat all your body needs to fuel itself—all you want. But you must learn to stop eating when you feel satisfied, and feel satisfied when you no longer feel hunger—not when you are stuffed. You should eat six to nine small meals a day—eat less, more often. You never have to go hungry.

Most important of all, eat as much of your food as possible raw.

Cooking destroys foods' enzymes, which are important catalysts for biochemical reactions all over the body. The more enzymes you provide your body with, the less energy it needs to expend on all those myriad functions.

Foods you do cook, you should heat for as short a time as possible, and preferably to no more than 118 degrees Fahrenheit.

LET'S GET SPIRITUAL

As you start eating a more alkaline diet, you will experience physical change. That's the main idea, after all, with the main change you're aiming for being bidding diabetes good riddance. But you should know that as you change for the better physically, you'll be improving psychologically as well; one feeds right into the other, on a two-way street. As you grow both physically and emotionally stronger, you'll think better, and you'll do better—and you'll be able to connect to your true self. And that, my friends, is spirituality, though it may come in a thousand disguises. This is the key to ultimate health, fitness, energy, vitality, love, joy, and happiness.

That's just one more way to say: Eat your veggies! I promised you it wasn't complicated. But of course, there are a few guidelines you need to know to set your course. This chapter explains the basic principles in some more detail in the hope that understanding their importance will ease the journey for you. The facts should motivate you when the going gets tough. Knowledge will set you free.

ELIMINATE SUGAR

Cut out all foods that contain moderate or high levels of sugars. That would include most fruits and fruit juices, grains, starchy vegetables like potatoes, yams, and corn, and dairy products, as well as anything with added sugars, including "natural" sugars such as honey and maple syrup. Your body makes no distinction in how it reacts to various kinds of sugars; they all raise your blood glucose level and thus the acidity of your blood and tissues.

Americans consume more than a third of a pound of sugar each day! Diabetes cases have more than tripled since 1958; our sugar consumption has risen similarly. You don't need me to connect the dots for you, do you? Sugar consumption correlates with obesity as well. To take just one example, recent studies show that drinking one sugar-sweetened soda a day increases the risk of obesity by 60 percent in children and adolescents (and not to unduly scare you or anything, but about 65 percent of teen girls and 74 percent of teen boys get that soda-a-day).

A NATURAL SWEETENER THAT WON'T RAISE YOUR BLOOD SUGAR

Stevia is an herbal sweetener you can find at your health food store. It is intensely sweet and all natural, and won't raise your blood sugar levels. It's even got quite a track record as a treatment of Type 2 diabetes, and may be helpful in reducing dependence on supplemental insulin. Scientists have shown it to be safe—noncarcinogenic—too. And it's nutritious, containing various vitamins and minerals, including vitamin A, rutin, zinc, magnesium, and iron. All in all, the sooner you switch to it from sugar or artificial sweeteners, the better!

Other studies show stevia can lower blood pressure, decrease the incidence of colds and flus, suppress tobacco and alcohol cravings, and reduce appetite (helping with weight loss). It's also been used to treat systemic yeast infections and even, topically, skin cancer.

It's the effect on diabetes that's most important here, however. Holistic doctors have used stevia to regulate blood sugar levels for many years. Try taking it in droplet form with meals to bring blood sugar levels to near normal.

Two recent studies on rats and mice in Denmark showed that a stevia extract brought blood sugar levels into the normal range. Work coming out of Brazil looked at volunteers who took a glucose tolerance test. Those also given stevia extracts had significantly lower blood sugar levels than those who didn't.

A sugar by any other name may or may not be just as sweet, but it is definitely just as bad for you. So look out for: corn syrup, dextrin, dextrose, dulcitol, fructose, glucose, honey, lactose, levulose, maltose, mannitol, mannose, molasses, saccharose, sorbitol, sorghum, treacle, turbinado, xylitol, and xylose. Remember, anything ending in an -*ose* is a sugar (though not all sugars end in -*ose*). Also steer clear of artificial sugars such as saccharin and aspartame, including Sweet'N Low, Equal, Sweet One, and Sugar Twin. These are usually 96 percent glucose and 4 percent artificial sweeteners. Artificial sweeteners can ferment into acids—including formaldehyde—that are devastating to your pancreas and insulin-producing beta cells.

DOES THIS HAVE SUGAR IN IT?

If you are unsure whether or not something contains sugar, you can test it with a Clinistix or Keto-Diastix (though they don't work on dairy products). Whatever you're testing must be liquid, so you may have to do some pureeing or juicing—or chewing!—first. You can get Clinistix or Diastix at most pharmacies. The lightest color on the test strip indicates a very low concentration of sugar. You can also use Clinistix or Diastix to test sugar levels in your urine.

LIMIT CARBOHYDRATES

Your body promptly turns even complex carbohydrates into sugars, so stick with low-carbohydrate foods. Your focus should be mainly on green vegetables, largely forsaking grains such as wheat, rice, barley, oats, and especially corn, as well as the cereals, pastas, pastries, and myriad other foods made with them. Yes, I know this flies in the face of that famous USDA food pyramid, with its wide base of bread, cereal, rice, and pasta. All I can say is, I believe that pyramid is a recipe for disaster for anyone, and especially diabetics. It's a setup for bombarding your body with sugars, in the fast lane to overacidity.

Think about it: When cattle ranchers want to fatten up their livestock for slaughter, they put them on a diet almost exclusively made up of grains that would definitely get the thumbs-up from the designers of that pyramid. The sugars in those grains (maltose) ferment into acids, and the cows make body fat to bind the acids to preserve their pH balance. If they lived long enough, those would be some Type 2 diabetic cows.

Any extra sugars in the body, from carbs to any other sugars, that aren't needed right away for cellular energy will be fermented by bacteria and yeast, creating an increase in acidity of the body. But when you reduce carbs and all sugars, you will not only reduce sugar levels, and acidity, but also lower cholesterol levels.

NO-NOS

To keep your body in pH balance, you must be careful to avoid:

- Acidic drinks such as coffee, black tea, and soda. Caffeine is an acid, and it signals the body to hop on board the blood sugar level roller coaster. Decaf coffee is just as bad, because the decaffeinating process adds two acids to the mix—one being formaldehyde.
- Alcohol (an acid), including beer and wine.

- Chocolate. Besides caffeine, chocolate contains two other toxic acids.
- Mushrooms and other edible fungi, and algae.
- Yeast, both baker's and brewer's.
- Malted products.
- Fermented or aged foods and condiments, including soy sauce, vinegar, and MSG (and anything made with soy sauce, vinegar, or MSG, such as salad dressings or marinades), sauerkraut, yogurt, miso, tempeh, olives, pickles, horseradish, tamari, mayonnaise, mustard, ketchup, steak sauce, and barbecue sauce.

DAIRY

I believe a diet rich in dairy products is one of the leading causes of diabetes. Consider Finland: It has both the world's highest level of consumption of cow's milk—and the highest incidence of Type 1 diabetes. A 1992 study published in the *New England Journal of Medicine* compared Finnish children who were diabetic to those who weren't, and found levels of antibodies to certain cow's milk proteins to be *seven times higher* in the diabetic kids. A French study got similar results, and also found high levels of those antibodies in a fifth of children with prediabetes.

A 1984 study clearly linked diet and diabetes when it followed people in Western Samoa and Singapore, communities with almost no Type 1 diabetes, as they moved to Australia or New Zealand. Rates of diabetes skyrocketed in one or two generations, quickly matching those of native Aussies and New Zealanders. Of all the environmental factors that changed in the lives of these immigrants, diet was most clearly suspect. The case for the Samoans was particularly dramatic. Two mainstays of the Western diet are strikingly scarce in Western Samoa: wheat—and cow's milk.

More evidence for the dairy–diabetes link comes from the youngest humans. Several studies, both epidemiological and clinical, show that exclusive breast-feeding (and therefore a delayed exposure to infant formula, most of which is based on cow's milk) reduces the risk of diabetes. The longer babies are breast-fed, and the later their first exposure to formula comes, the lower their risk of diabetes.

Eating excessive amounts of dairy products overloads the body with lactose—a sugar, after all—which calls for more insulin and starting that whole vicious cycle. Fermented by yeast, lactose creates a buildup of lactic acid in the body. To bring your body back into alkaline balance, you're going to have to eliminate dairy products.

Joel's Story

I was recently diagnosed with Type 2 diabetes. I had a fasting blood sugar of 178, and it soared to 345 two hours after I ate breakfast. I decided to try the pH Miracle program for controlling diabetes. I'd already been taking 1 liter of green drink a day, and now I added supplements for pancreas and adrenal support, 1 tablespoon of each, three times a day. I also took chromium, vanadium, vitamin C, and calcium.

I also upgraded my diet, learning to avoid sugar and carbohydrates, and became a regular at my local health food store. I started to read labels on foods more than ever before. I switched from oatmeal to a buckwheat cereal for breakfast, and from milk to soy milk. I cut out all dairy products and bought yeast-free bread and rye crackers. I have always eaten lots of vegetables, but I upped the amount even more. What is amazing is that with all the great recipes, I don't miss the old way of eating at all. The secret is that the food is interesting, colorful, and tasteful.

Within two months of beginning the program, I dropped 26 pounds; only 6 more to go to get to 200, the same weight I was in my college athletics days. My fasting blood sugar level was tested to be 111. My doctor was amazed at such fast and dramatic improvement. I knew I had experienced a real pH miracle for myself.

MEAT

Remember those grain-fattened cows? They don't live long enough (because they are slaughtered for food) to suffer from the problems that their diet would create for them, but they pass all the acid built up in their muscles and fat along to you when you eat them. Even without that last blast of carbs, animal foods form lots of acids as they are digested. Meat is hard to digest, taking up to an entire day, long enough for it to rot in the digestive tract. (That's disgusting enough on its own, but remember that this also means the meat is acidifying.) Up to half the body's energy expenditure can be drained off in the service of digesting animal proteins.

Because of the way meat animals are raised, slaughtered, and aged in the United States, meat also often has high levels of bacteria, yeast, and fungi, as well as associated toxins and acids. Meat "aged" for human consumption is actually partially fermented, and as such will be permeated with acids and acid-generating microforms. The

---

STILL TEMPTED?

If you need any more reasons to avoid meat, let me add to your list. Meat (and animal protein in general) is:

- High in cholesterol.
- Typically laden with antibiotics and hormones.
- Linked to increased risk of cancer, heart disease, colitis, obesity, and many other diseases, not the least of which is diabetes.
- Hard on the environment. It takes two hundred times the land and ten times the water to produce 1 pound of beef as it does to yield 1 pound of avocado or other plant food; grazing causes soil depletion and erosion and in some places requires deforestation; animal wastes (including gas) pollute the air, land, and water.

uric acid produced in the process was proven to induce diabetes in animals in studies dating back to 1954; the sulfuric acid formed has similar effects. In 1989, scientists documented that animals' feed was a major source of toxins in meat animals—microform wastes found in corn, peanuts, cottonseed, barley, oats, and wheat show up in edible animal tissue. And the toxins were found to be heat-resistant—that is, they didn't go away during cooking! Furthermore, diets high in animal protein can lead to an increase in blood sugars.

Humans are not designed to be carnivores anyway. Our digestive tract is long and complicated, meant for the slow absorption of complex and stable plant food. True carnivores have short, simple bowels, for minimum transit time. They also have different intestinal flora than humans. Not to mention teeth and jaws meant for tearing apart animal flesh.

WHAT TO EAT

All that said, I don't want to belabor the things you shouldn't eat. More important is the glory of nature's bounty in providing foods to truly nourish every cell in your body. This next section, then, gives you an overview of your healthiest choices of what to put in your body. Always choose whole, natural, organic, unprocessed, unrefined foods. And eat them raw as much as possible.

EAT FAT

Yes, fat. What "everyone knows" about eating a low-fat diet for heart health is wrong. At least, partially wrong. It's true that eating too much saturated and partially hydrogenated fat isn't good for you. They aren't the real culprits, however, or at least they don't act alone. It's the nutritional poverty of the diet they are a part of—rich only in sugar and unhealthy fats—that's the real problem. Fat and oil aren't, on their own, anything bad. The truth is, your body absolutely needs fats for good health. Fats are necessary for making hormones, cushioning joints and protecting muscles, buffering acids, stimulating the brain, making cell membranes, and fueling the body. A low-fat diet is dangerous! You must, however, choose your fats wisely. *Good* fats will be the most important food you eat to regulate and control your blood sugar and insulin.

Monounsaturated fat is important in reversing diabetes. Take olive oil as a prime example: A study published in the *Journal of the American Medical Association* in 1994 followed forty-two Type 2 patients for almost six months and found that a diet higher in olive oil/monounsaturated fat reduced blood sugar, insulin, and triglycerides as compared to a diet low in fat and high in carbs. The mainline American Diabetes Association also recommends a diet rich in monounsaturated fats to improve glucose tolerance and reduce insulin resistance for better control of diabetes. Monounsaturated fat binds with acid to protect the body, including the heart and blood vessels.

The best sources of monounsaturated fat are olive oil, raw nuts, and avocado. Monounsaturated fats won't break down into transfatty acids (see below) when heated, so they are your best bet when lightly "steam-frying" vegetables or fish. Most of the benefits of olive oil are removed when it is refined, so be sure to get cold-pressed, virgin olive oil. It provides beta-carotene and vitamin E (both excellent buffers of gastrointestinal and metabolic acids), along with a host of lesser-known health promoters with such jobs as forming healthy red blood cells, limiting the absorption of cholesterol from food, reducing inflammation, stimulating the flow of bile to help alkalize food coming out of the stomach, producing fat-digesting enzymes, and lowering the amount of circulating cholesterol.

The fats you must avoid are saturated fats (in meats and dairy products) and, more deadly, trans-fatty acids, aka trans fats. Trans fats are vegetable oils artificially kept solid at room temperature, such as those in shortening and margarine. This is what's meant by "partially hydrogenated vegetable oils" on food labels. Trans fats are used to cook most french fries and other fast foods, as well as in commercial baked goods, where they act as preservatives. Trans fats increase LDL and decrease HDL, with twice as bad an effect on the ratio between the two as saturated fat. I believe our increasing consumption of trans fats is behind the current epidemic of heart disease.

Polyunsaturated fats such as flax, borage, evening primrose, grape seed, and hemp oils are good, too. The other good fats you must know about are essential fatty acids (EFAs). The name comes from the fact that they are essential to human health, but must come through diet (or supplements) because the human body can't make them itself.

You get EFAs primarily from fish oils and a variety of seed oils. The two main types of omega-3s are EPA (eicosapentaenoic acid) and DHA (docasahexaenoic acid), found in cold-water fish. ALA (alpha-linolenic acid), which the body converts into EPA and then DHA, can be found in plant sources. It can be stored in the body until it is needed. (EPA and DHA are not stored.) The two main types of omega-6s are LA (linoleic acid) and GLA (gamma-linolenic acid), and come from certain plants.

EFAs perform many beneficial services in the body. Prime among them, from the diabetic's point of view, is their ability to bind and neutralize acid in the blood, and increase metabolic rate (helping with weight loss). EFAs are helpful in treating nerve degeneration in Type 2 diabetes. My own work has shown that taking EFAs can even decrease the amount of insulin diabetics require.

Omega-3s and 6s are required for building the membranes of all cells in the body. EFAs also lubricate joints, insulate the body against heat loss, and prevent skin from drying out. They lower the risk of heart attack and stroke by lowering arteriosclerosis, triglycerides, total cholesterol, LDL, and blood clots (including the blood clots that can cause gangrene and blindness in diabetics). The body needs EFAs to make prostaglandins, and prostaglandins are critical to many hormonal actions, inflammatory responses, and chromosome stability. Animal studies indicate that EFAs can inhibit the growth and metastasis of tumors. A study that followed newly diagnosed diabetics for five years found that the half of the group that received a diet enriched with LA had fewer cardiovascular problems than those who remained on a typical American diet. Wider-ranging studies have established that Inuit have an extremely low incidence of heart disease and strokes, despite their extremely fatty diet—fats derived mainly from fish and chock-full of EFAs. Because diabetics so often have dangerous high cholesterol and triglycerides, they should take heart (pun intended) from studies like the one done at the Oregon Health Sciences University, which showed that patients given supplementary fish oil for four weeks had, on average, a 46 percent drop in cholesterol (from 373 to 207)—and an even more dramatic drop in triglycerides, from 1,353 mg/dl to 281.

The typical American diet does not contain much in the way of omega-3s. The best source is fish. ALA is found in flaxseed, hemp, walnut, and soybean oils; your best bet is flaxseed oil, which is 57 percent ALA (and about 16 percent omega-6s to boot). Omega-6s, on the other hand, are easily obtained, because they're found in more commonly consumed vegetable oils, nuts, and seeds, including sunflower and sesame seeds and oils. Still, the best sources are out of the ordinary: borage, evening primrose, hemp, and black currant, in addition to sunflower oil. Borage seed oil contains up to 24 percent GLA, more than twice as much as evening primrose, for perspective, and also about 34 percent LA.

Your body requires a balance between omega-3s and omega-6s. Many experts consider three parts omega-6 to one part omega-3 to be the ideal for intake. The ratio in the brain is about 1:1, in the fat tissue, about 5:1; and in other tissue, about 4:1. A ratio of 3:1 in what you eat will support those ratios. Hemp oil comes the closest to reproducing this on its own, because it contains three parts omega-6 for each part omega-3. The typical American diet, however, is hugely lopsided, providing a ratio of twenty or thirty to one.

I recommend to all my non-vegetarian patients that they eat fresh fish several times a week, and that's absolutely crucial for people with diabetes. Choose fresh (not farm-raised) fish, fatty ones like salmon, mackerel, trout, sardines, tuna, eel, halibut, and swordfish. Besides being so rich in EFAs, fish is also an excellent low-acid source of all essential amino acids, vitamins A and D, several B vitamins, and many minerals, including calcium and potassium, and trace minerals including fluoride, iodine, zinc, and iron.

You should also use olive oil, flax oil, flax meal, and other EFA-rich oils, and mixed oils such as the essential oils available from Barlean's and Udo's, regularly, on steamed veggies, in soups, and as salad dressings—1 to 2 tablespoons a day. Select unrefined, expeller-pressed oils, and keep them away from heat, light, and even air to prevent rancidity (which not only makes them taste bad, but also reduces their beneficial properties). Eat nuts and seeds, especially almonds, hazelnuts, walnuts, and pecans, and sesame, flax and sunflower seeds, unsalted, and raw rather than roasted. (Avoid peanuts, however, which get rancid very quickly and are generally full of yeast and mold.) You can enjoy nut "milks," too, like almond milk, as long as they are unsweetened. And eat plenty of avocado, at least one a day for every 50 pounds of body weight. You can also take EFA supplements, about which more information appears in the next chapter. Healthy fats in your diet should account for 40 to 65 percent of your calories each day.

I believe people with diabetes are suffering from an EFA deficiency. High blood sugar makes EFAs in fat tissues unavailable to the body. My studies indicate that liberal amounts of EFAs in the diet—60 g or 2 ounces a day—make a dramatic difference in how much oral or injectable insulin diabetes patients need.

BEST SOURCES OF GOOD FAT IN YOUR FOOD

- Fish
- Nuts
- Seeds
- Avocado
- Coconut oil
- Healthy oils

WATER

The best way to get acid out of your body is to wash it out. The best way to wash it out is to provide plenty of water to do the job.

The human body is made primarily of water: It is 70 percent water, to be exact. Water makes up 70 percent of muscles, 25 percent of fats, 75 percent of the brain, and more than 80 percent of the blood. Water regulates body temperature, cushions and protects vital organs, aids in digestion, transports nutrients within cells—and dispels acidic wastes. You simply can't live without it. You can go a lot longer without food than you can without water. Even mild dehydration can cause impaired concentration, headaches, irritability, fatigue, and lethargy. Maintaining proper hydration is critical to the health of your pancreas as well as the health of your body as a whole.

But you need not just water, but the right kind of water. You need to start with clean, uncontaminated water, of course. The water should also be alkaline. To ensure both, it should be purified, distilled, or perhaps even ionized, reduced, or micro-ionized. (More about that in a moment.) Ideally, you'd drink pure rainwater, or water just emerged from a spring. The farther from its source it gets and the more it runs through open country, impure environments, sources of pollution, or just distribution pipes, the more acidic water becomes, the more impurities become dissolved in it, and the more electrons it loses.

This last item is given little attention, but it is crucially important. The more electrons water has, the more energy it contains. The more energy it contains, the more energy it can bring to your body. Water with lots of electrons (called, unfortunately, "reduced" water, due to an early scientific misunderstanding about the flow of electrical current) counters oxidative stress—the same thing that makes antioxidant vitamins so important. Furthermore, acids are saturated with protons (positively charged particles), which negatively charged electrons bind to and neutralize.

Most common sources of water are highly oxidized (low in electrons), and the body has to add huge amounts of electrons to even it out with the levels of electrons needed in the blood—then promptly loses those electrons as they are passed out of the body as urine. This is especially acute in diabetics, because they not only make excess urine, but are also so acidic that their urine is often loaded with electrons bound to acids' protons. This is an enormous drain on energy reserves, and places a lot of stress on the pancreas (among other things).

Recent studies from Norway published in the journal *Diabetes Care* suggest a link between acidic drinking water and Type 1 diabetes. Researchers evaluated tap-water samples from the homes of more than three hundred children, and found that children whose water was acidic were more than three and a half times as likely to be diagnosed with diabetes compared to those with less acidic drinking water.

Since most of us don't have easy access to fresh mountain spring-water straight from the source, your best bet is water that has been purified through reverse osmosis filtration or distillation, then put through the process of electromagnetic micro-ionization to add electrons. Be sure to use a reservoir-type device where the water is exposed to direct current for several minutes to collect electrons; the flow-through machines (fitted directly to the cold-water tap and dispensing water immediately) don't allow enough time for the water to be charged. (See the resources section.) I know this sounds difficult, but all you really need is the right equipment. Then it is no more complicated than filling a typical water filter pitcher: Just fill the purifier/ionizer, let it run—and drink up! If you refill and run it each time you empty it, you'll have healthful water ready to come out of the spigot any time you need it.

Adults lose, on average, about 10 cups—roughly 2.5 liters—of water every day through sweating, exhaling, urinating, and bowel movements. Very active people lose even more, and most diabetics lose in excess of 4 liters a day in removing excess acids. At the very least, then, you need to replace what you're losing. Radiant health requires more liquid, however. If you're only drinking enough to cover your losses, you won't provide enough water to flush out all those acids. However you look at it, surveys continue to show that Americans are simply not drinking enough.

Vegetables are about 90 percent water, so a plant-based diet like the pH Miracle plan will go a long way toward keeping you hydrated. Still, you should be drinking at least 4 liters of alkaline, energized water a day. I've seen clients get results with as little as 1 liter a day of water prepared as described in this section, but you won't reap all the benefits you otherwise might. It is, however, a sensible place to start for many people, increasing how much you drink gradually, to make this a change you can live with—for life.

Make sure your water is alkaline, with a pH of 8.0 or above, by adding 16 drops per liter of 2 percent sodium chlorite or sodium silicate to distilled water (see chapter 7). Better still: Add powdered greens, 1 teaspoon per liter, and perhaps powdered soy sprouts as well, 1 teaspoon per liter. This is what I call a "green drink." Some fresh lemon juice helps as well—with alkalinity as well as taste. You could also juice vegetables, and drink that mixed in a 1:10 ratio with water. If you need to get rid of acid quickly, you could also use 10 g (3 teaspoons) of sodium bicarbonate (baking soda) in 1 liter of distilled water.

Kimberly's Story

I've struggled for almost twenty years with my Type 1 diabetes to attain normalcy in my blood sugar readings. Along the way I've tried a variety of regimes, but it has always been a losing battle. When I stuck with the traditional food pyramid, I kept consistently normal levels only by exercising myself to exhaustion. I've tried vegetarianism, yoga, eating by ayurvedic principles, and a host of herbs and vitamins touted as helping blood sugar regularity. No matter what I did, I always had unquenchable cravings for more food, healthy and otherwise, and time and again I'd slide out of my routine, then suffer higher and higher blood sugar readings as a result. I certainly never believed there was a way to cure my diabetes.

I had all but given up when I investigated the pH Miracle program not for me, but for my husband, hoping the focus on reducing acid would bring him some relief from the horrendous acid indigestion he's suffered with for most of his life. To my surprise, after eating and drinking in this balanced way for just a short time, my blood sugar was often low, and I was needing to eat more and more in order to maintain the level of insulin I was on. (I've often wondered at the fact that insulin—in the case of insulin reactions—is more life threatening than diabetes itself, at least in the immediate sense.) It finally hit me: Why not lower my insulin dose, rather than eating more than I needed/wanted? To someone who has been diabetic for two decades, the idea seemed preposterous—and miraculous. By five months on the program, I'd cut my insulin by more than half, while experiencing consistently normal to low blood sugar readings, day after day. I had no trace of microalbumin in my urine, either, though I always did until I started this program. What's more, my cholesterol went down to 177, from 233. My weight didn't change much—I always tend to stay around my ideal anyway—but I no longer had so many of those physical cravings for foods harmful to my body (though I'll admit I fought them for a while). At last I decided to try a liquid feast, and after a few days my blood sugar readings were entirely normal—with no insulin at all! I'm hopeful I've seen the last of those injections.

Besides all that, my husband did indeed have no indigestion whatsoever while eating and drinking this way—and he lost 15 pounds to boot!

This isn't complicated—simply eating the healthiest foods, raw, leafy vegetables and pure water being the highlights, and eating when I'm hungry, and eating until I feel satisfied—but it hasn't been easy. I realize, however, that my health—my life!—is in my own hands. It has required all the willpower and discipline I have—and then some—but I have wrought my own miracle and what could be more wonderful than that? I'd pay any price for what I have received: no more worries about physical health, and the promise of living wisely and well until the day I die. I am eternally grateful for this program, and the way it has transformed my life.

VEGETABLES

Joining healthy fats as the foundation for the new house of health you're building are vegetables, particularly green vegetables. Vegetables are generally low in calories, low in sugar, and rich in nutrients. Just about all the vitamins, minerals, and micronutrients your body needs can be found in vegetables, which can also provide macronutrients such as protein and (healthy) fats. They offer lots of fiber, which regulates digestion and helps soak up acids, as well as alkalinizing salts that neutralize acids and protect against microform overgrowth. Vegetables are an excellent source of enzymes, while the phytonutrients that give plants color (like yellow and orange) also neutralize acids and help prevent diabetes, cardiovascular disease, obesity, high cholesterol, and more.

You must avoid the handful of vegetables that form acid upon digestion, but by and large eating your veggies is key to keeping your body alkaline and your blood sugar levels balanced.

Make vegetables the majority of the food on your plate. Concentrate on all the green veggies that grow above the ground. Eat all you

QUICK FIXES FOR LOW BLOOD SUGAR

There is one time when the sugar in starchy vegetables can come in handy: if your blood sugar levels drop below 50 mg/dl and you need to raise them quickly. Don't reach for the ultimately devastating juice or candy bar that may have been recommended to you by traditional doctors. Instead, reach for an all-natural solution:

- Have a glass of fresh almond milk (see page 183).
- Snack on a carrot, beet, or red or new potato, or have a fresh vegetable juice with some carrot or beet juice added (be sure to dilute the juice 1:10 in pure water). You could also add a teaspoon of green powder and pH drops.
- Eat a bowl of tomato and avocado chunks with broccoli.
- Drink a glass of AvoRado Kid Super Green Shake (see page 177).
- Take 1 tablespoon of soy sprouts powder and chase it with 1 liter of green drink with pH drops.

want of low-carbohydrate green vegetables such as spinach, broccoli, celery, kale, cucumber, leafy greens, avocado, and green peppers. To broaden your palate, you'll also want to get plenty of red, orange, and yellow peppers, and tomatoes. The universe of vegetables is one of wonderful variety, and you should eat freely of all but a few. (Exceptions include legumes—except sprouted; see below—and sugary root vegetables: carrots, beets, potatoes, and sweet potatoes). I want to take some time now to look more closely at a few of the superstars.

Avocados

Avocados are actually an oily berry fruit, but I'm listing them here because most people consider them a vegetable. Either way, they are just about the perfect food. They are full of protein and healthy, monounsaturated fats (which give them their rich, smooth texture and flavor). They are also full of fiber and water, which help the body clear out acids. Avocados are quickly digested, so they don't putrefy in the stomach or intestines the way animal fats and proteins do, and they create twice as much usable energy as they require to be digested. And avocados have an alkalizing effect in the blood and tissues as they are metabolized, yet contain no starch and very little sugar, so they do not raise blood sugar levels.

Furthermore, avocados are chockablock with chemical compounds that lower cholesterol (phytosterol), buffer acids (glutathione), and protect against cataracts, macular degeneration, and certain types of cancer (lutein)—up to three or four times as much as found in other common vegetables and fruits. Avocados contain fourteen minerals, including iron and copper and more potassium and sodium than bananas, without all the sugar. Avocados are also one of the best sources of vitamin E.

For all these reasons, avocado will be one of the most important foods to eat as your body moves away from sugar metabolism to fat metabolism. My research shows that eating liberal amounts of avocado helps in normalizing blood sugar levels. I recommend eating three to five a day.

CARING FOR AVOCADOS

Avocados ripen after they are picked; allow four to seventeen days for softening, depending on the variety, ambient temperature, and humidity. Keep your avocados out on the table or counter, and pinch the tops and bottoms each morning; when they yield to pressure on both ends, they are ripe. Refrigerate the ones you are not ready to eat. Keep prepared avocado in the refrigerator, wrapped in plastic to preserve freshness.

Tomatoes

Tomatoes, too, are technically fruit, though we commonly categorize them as vegetables. They are very low in sugar and help remove acids, especially the uric and sulfuric acid formed from meats, from the body. Tomatoes cleanse the liver, too, so it can keep doing its job clearing waste from the body.

Processed tomatoes, such as canned or bottled sauces or juice, are acidic, but fresh tomatoes are alkaline when they enter the bloodstream.

Broccoli

This vegetable contains cancer-fighting compounds, according to mainstream research at Johns Hopkins University and other labs. Broccoli is a great source of vitamin C—you get 97 percent of the recommended daily allowance in just 1 ounce—better than any citrus fruit. You also get folate, vitamin A, potassium, vitamin B_6, magnesium, and riboflavin. My own research has shown that broccoli and broccoli sprouts chelate metabolic acids; provide chlorophyll for cellular cleansing; and provide glucoraphanin, which acts as an anti-acid in the blood and tissues. Broccoli lowers and/or balances blood sugars, lowers cholesterol, and helps in weight loss, among other things. So eat hearty—and look for broccoli as an ingredient in your green drink.

Cucumbers

Cukes are low in sugar and high in potassium, and they contain plenty of water, making them one of the best alkalizing agents you can have. I recommend cucumbers rather than carrots as a base for juicing, to avoid all the sugar in carrots. Cucumbers are cooling, especially when used in juices or in water, and can even be used in a bath to draw acids out through the skin. Among several beneficial phytochemicals, cucumbers contain monoterpenes, which help reduce and neutralize gastrointestinal and metabolic acids, as well as cutting production of cholesterol.

Onion and Garlic

Along with jicama and ginger, onions and garlic represent the beneficial root vegetables. Garlic and onions work to significantly lower blood sugar, thanks to their allicin and allyl propyl disulfide (APDS) content. Their flavonoids probably help as well. APDS and allicin help increase insulin, lowering blood sugar.

Onions help metabolize glucose, increase insulin, and/or prevent the destruction of insulin. Research has shown that the more onion you take in, the more your blood sugar will be lowered, but beneficial effects are seen even at levels low enough to be a normal part of your diet.

Onions and garlic also have cardiovascular benefits that are even more important to people with diabetes. They lower cholesterol and blood pressure, and prevent the buildup of plaque in your arteries. On top of all that, onions and garlic contain a large amount of sulfur and are good acid buffers, so they'll help you maintain a healthy pH balance in your body.

Wheatgrass and Barley Grass

These grasses are good for you for all the reasons all green vegetables are excellent choices, but they get their own little section here because they are also an excellent source of protein—more than meat, poultry, fish, or eggs. This is the secret of some of the strongest, most muscled animals in the world. Elephants, gorillas, bears, horses, cows—all herbivores. All grass eaters.

Grasses are some of the lowest-calorie, lowest-sugar, most nutrient-rich foods on the planet. Wheatgrass contains more than a hundred nutrients, including every identified mineral and trace mineral and all the B vitamins, including B_{12}, which is usually considered to be available only from animal sources. It is rich in vitamins C, E, and K, and has one of the highest levels of vitamin A of any food. Plus, it is 25 percent protein and has high amounts of an antifungal/antimycotoxin called laetrile. Barley grass has seven times more vitamin C than oranges and four times as much thiamine (vitamin B_1) as whole wheat flour—thirty times as much as milk. Grasses contain more iron than spinach.

Grasses help balance blood sugar levels; just 3 ounces of juiced wheat- or barley grass in a liter of distilled water will normalize high or low blood sugar in fifteen minutes. In addition, grasses are natural buffers of metabolic acids.

But perhaps the most powerful of grass's elements is its chlorophyll—the "blood" of the plant. Chlorophyll helps human blood deliver oxygen throughout the body. It cuts down on acids binding to DNA, and breaks down calcium oxalate to help neutralize and dispose of excess acid.

The molecular structure of chlorophyll is nearly identical to that of the hemoglobin (an oxygen transporter) in human blood. Both are composed of the same four elements—carbon, hydrogen, oxygen, and nitrogen—though hemoglobin is organized around a single iron atom, while chlorophyll is organized around a single magnesium atom. I believe that chlorophyll helps build healthy blood cells, regenerating our bodies at the molecular and cellular levels.

Chlorophyll is what makes plants green, and all green plants (veggies) have it. The two best sources for humans are wheatgrass and barley grass. The best way to include them in your diet is not through eating them as is (leave that to the cud-chewing cows), but to juice them to extract and condense their healing power for your body's use.

Spinach

Spinach is another wonder vegetable you should be sure appears often on your plate, as well as in your green drink. It is rich in vitamin A, folate, iron, magnesium, calcium, vitamin C, riboflavin, potassium, and vitamin B_6, not to mention being a great source of fiber. Spinach helps improve blood pressure and cholesterol levels, aids in losing weight, and generally helps reduce acid in the body, fighting diabetes (along with much else).

Soybeans

Soybeans are another great source of protein—more than fish, eggs, or dairy products—without cholesterol or saturated fat. They have the distinction of being the only vegetable to contain all of the eight essential amino acids used to make proteins. Considered a complete food because of that, along with their carbohydrate and fat content, soybeans also provide an impressive array of minerals and vitamins, including calcium, iron, phosphorus, magnesium, thiamine, riboflavin, niacin, and even B_{12} (normally thought to come only from animal foods). In addition, soybeans provide both omega-3 and omega-6 EFAs. Soybeans also contain many powerful beneficial phytochemicals—like the isoflavones you may have been hearing about—with cancer-fighting potential.

That's why soy is such an important part of the pH miracle plan for diabetes. You do have to steer clear of fermented soy products—miso, tempeh, soy sauce, tamari—but edamame (whole soybeans), tofu, and soy sprouts (more about them coming right up) should make regular appearances on your menus. Soybean oil and lecithin are good choices, too. Most soy milk is sweetened by rice syrup, but if you can find (and like) unsweetened soy milk, that makes a good addition as well.

Sprouts

These are among the very best foods you can eat. They have all the nutrients of the full-grown plant within them, but concentrated and energized with the spark of life, so each tiny package is literally bursting with good stuff—thirty to fifty times the concentration of nutrients found in mature plants. Sprouts are filled with vitamins (including vitamin B_{12}, found mostly in animal sources), minerals, and complete proteins, and are high in enzymes and nucleic acids. Alfalfa sprouts contains 7 g of protein per 1-ounce serving, for example, and if you dehydrate soy sprouts (as in the soy sprouts powder in a green drink) to concentrate the proteins, fats, and minerals even further, you get twenty to thirty times what you get in the sprouts themselves. Sprouts are packed with plant compounds that aid digestion and promote cellular organization, and they are alkaline forming on digestion. The protein and fats in sprouts are broken down into easily assimilated amino acids and fatty acids, and their starches are broken down into gentle vegetable sugars that do not raise blood sugar levels.

You can grow sprouts in your own kitchen from beans, lentils, grains, seeds, and nuts for fresh organic produce in any season. Or, of course, you can buy them. Eat sprouts on their own, or in salads, or gently steamed with other veggies, or sprinkled over soup. Start with bean, mung, broccoli, soy, radish, and sunflower sprouts. Whichever and however you like them, you should eat them every day.

NUTRITIONAL VALUES OF VEGETABLES AND SPROUTS

These veggies support the pancreas, help lower blood glucose and cholesterol, assist with weight loss, and provide fiber to neutralize systemic acid. Obviously we don't have space to cover every last alkaline vegetable, but this sampling of nutrition facts will give you an idea of why they are great to eat on their own, or to have in a green drink.

ALKALINE VEGETABLE NUTRITION	
Vegetable	% of RDA in a 1-ounce serving
Alfalfa sprouts	Folate: 3%
Broccoli	Vitamin C: 97% Folate: 20% Vitamin A: 11% Iron: 7% Potassium: 6% Vitamin B$_6$: 6% Magnesium: 5% Riboflavin: 5%
Dandelion greens	Vitamin A: 61% Vitamin C: 16% Calcium: 9% Iron: 9% Riboflavin: 5%
Kale	Vitamin C: 57% Iron: 13% Vitamin A: 13% Calcium: 11% Magnesium: 11% Potassium: 5%
Kelp	Folate: 25% Magnesium: 10% Iron: 8% Calcium: 6%
Okra	Vitamin C: 22% Folate: 18% Magnesium 13% Vitamin B$_6$: 8% Potassium: 7% Thiamin: 7% Calcium: 6%

Vegetable	% of RDA in a 1-ounce serving
Parsley	Vitamin C: 45% Folate: 27% Iron: 19% Vitamin A: 16%
Spinach	Vitamin A: 74% Folate: 66% Iron: 32% Magnesium: 22% Calcium: 15% Vitamin C: 15% Riboflavin: 12% Potassium: 11% Vitamin B_6: 11%
Tomato	Vitamin C: 39% Folate: 9% Vitamin A: 8% Potassium: 7% Iron: 6%
Watercress	Vitamin C: 12% Vitamin A: 8%
Oat grass	Thiamin: 9% Magnesium: 8% Iron: 6%
Soybean sprouts	Folate: 30% Vitamin C: 9% Thiamin: 8% Iron: 7% Magnesium: 7%
Celery	Folate: 8% Vitamin C: 7%
Cabbage	Vitamin C: 30% Folate: 8%

FRUIT

Most popular fruits are full of sugar, and therefore counterproductive on a diet meant to fight diabetes. But there are a few delicious exceptions.

Lemons, Limes, and Grapefruits

Despite seeming acidic, these citrus fruits become alkaline as they are digested, thanks to their potassium and sodium content. These low-sugar fruits do not significantly raise blood sugar, so you can eat them freely. Pink grapefruit has a little more sugar than white, but both are good choices. You can use lemon or lime juice, or unsweetened grapefruit juice, in any or all of your water/green drinks—it not only perks up the taste, but also helps balance your pH.

Coconuts

Coconuts have gotten a bad rap because of their high fat content. The fact of the matter is, however, that coconut is a great source of *good* fats, as well as proteins and minerals that help lower high blood sugars, reduce cholesterol, build healthy bones and blood, and provide fuel for the body's energy production.

True, processed coconut oils, having been refined and hydrogenated, hit you with deadly trans fats. But natural coconut is a whole different ball game.

Studies show that populations (such as those on tropical islands) that use a lot of coconut do *not* have increased risk of heart disease that would come with exposure to a lot of trans fats. They don't have high cholesterol, high rates of heart disease, or high death rates. Research on rats indicates that reliance on coconut fat had better effects on cholesterol levels than did sunflower oil. And when whole unsweetened coconut milk or coconut oil is added to an otherwise standard American diet, there is actually a small drop in cholesterol levels.

Coconut milk made by liquefying the white meat is a complete protein food when taken in its natural form. In fact, it is similar to breast milk in its chemical balance. It is an excellent source of phosphorus, calcium, and iron. Coconut contains antifungal compounds. It helps reduce acid, which in turn reduces the body's need for increased cholesterol to bind to the acid.

So go ahead, discover for yourself the benefits (not to mention deliciousness) of adding unsweetened organic coconut, coconut milk, and coconut oil to your diet. Try unsweetened flakes in your soups, on salads, or on fish.

SALT

Here's another chance to fly in the face of conventional wisdom: Make sure you get enough salt. That's a comical concept on the standard American diet, since processed and refined foods are very salty. But once you're on natural, organic foods exclusively, you'll also need to add some natural, organic salts or sodium. The body uses sodium to make potassium, and the balance between potassium and sodium at pretty high levels is important in maintaining pH balance. Salts (the right kinds, at least) strongly alkalize the body. Good health requires a sufficient (though reasonable) salt intake. The push for low-salt diets may sometimes make sense in addressing the typical American's diet, but current research reveals very few salt-related health problems. In fact, the biggest salt-related health problem is probably not getting enough!

In the form of sodium chloride, salt plays an important role in digestion and absorption of nutrients, activating the enzymes that begin the process, then generating hydrochloric acid in the stomach and releasing enzymatic and bile secretions from the gallbladder and pancreas to continue it. In the presence of salt, partially digested food is able to trigger some natural sodium bicarbonate, derived from sodium chloride, from the pancreas to buffer acids coming out of the stomach. Without salt, there can be no digestion.

We need not just sodium alone, however, but sodium in conjunction with the various minerals it interacts with, including chloride, chlorite, potassium, calcium, magnesium, silica, and hydrogen. So use liberal amounts of ocean salt, which contains plenty of minerals. You can buy it as Celtic Salt or RealSalt™.

YOU ARE WHAT YOU EAT. REALLY.

Making the right food choices is even more important than you might think, if you're conceiving of diabetes in the traditional medical sense and focusing on avoiding sugar. It's even more important than you might think if you're thinking somewhat more broadly and looking to counter the heart-endangering side effects that so often come with diabetes.

That's because our bodies are, quite literally, a biological transformation of the food we eat and the liquids we drink. We are truly becoming what we eat. In our gastrointestinal system, food is digested and absorbed as modern physiology describes, yes—but that is not the end of the story. In a final step, what we ingest is ultimately transformed into red blood cells.

Looking again to modern physiology, we'd learn that red blood cells carry oxygen to the cells and carbon dioxide (an acid) away from the cells. That's only part of it, however. Those red blood cells circulate throughout the body and transform themselves into body cells, such as liver, muscle, fat, brain, bones, heart, and, most to the point for this book, pancreatic and even insulin-producing beta cells. Red blood cells are the foundational material for every cell in our bodies.

To have healthy body cells, you have to have healthy red blood cells. To make healthy red blood cells, you need plenty of green foods and good fats. I have noted significant improvements in both the quality and quantity of red blood cells in my clients when they start living on high-chlorophyll foods and drinks and cellular-membrane-building good fats. To look at it through the lens of diabetes: Healthy pancreas and insulin-producing beta cells are determined by the quality and quantity of red blood cells, which is in turn determined by what you eat and drink. If you want a pancreas that functions properly, you have to build the blood and provide the proper alkaline environment.

A diet based on green foods and good fats will provide all your body needs to set this in motion. Microzymas organize themselves into amino acids. Cells select the specific amino acids they need and use them in construction of new blood cells, which become body cells (tissues and organs).

The key to preventing and reversing Type 1 and Type 2 diabetes and all their related symptoms is in the blood. The key to healthy blood is in the food. The key to good food is in you. All you have to do is choose health.

LISTEN TO WHAT THE EXPERTS SAY . . . AND DON'T DO IT

However minimal official dietary recommendations are—the famous food pyramid, the "5 a day" campaign to get you to eat fruits and veggies—most Americans still aren't living up to them. On average, 40 to 45 percent of our calories come from refined fat, and 20 to 25 percent from white sugar. Moreover, much of the remaining 30 to 40 percent comes from processed foods—canned or frozen veggies, frozen, processed meats, breads from refined flour, and so on. Most Americans get as little as 10 to 15 g of fiber a day, despite recommendations to get 30 to 60. The *Journal of the American Medical Association* reported in 2002 that although the average American diet may be sufficient to prevent vitamin deficiency diseases such as scurvy, the majority of Americans still have "suboptimal" levels of vitamins, putting them at increased risk of chronic diseases including diabetes as well as cardiovascular disease and cancer. There's no two ways about it: Our bodies are not getting what they need eating the way most of us eat. We take in excessive amounts of food (about 500 calories per day above recommendations, almost 900 calories per day more than the average twenty years ago), yet we are largely—and I do mean largely!—malnourished when it comes to what's needed to maintain good health.

We have to do better. But a lot of the experts aren't really helping. The USDA's food pyramid is deeply flawed, and with its emphasis on carbohydrates I believe it actually contributes to the onset of diabetes. Even the official guidelines from the American Diabetes

Association put the same emphasis on starches: The *Diabetes Food and Nutrition Bible* it publishes advises making starches "the centerpiece of the meal." Mainstream practitioners following the party line generally recommend that 45 to 60 percent of calories come from carbs (which, as I've mentioned, the body treats essentially the same as sugar). In fact, in 1994, the ADA announced that people with diabetes should follow the same dietary guidelines as anyone else, and that even sugar could be a part of their diet.

These people aren't crazy, of course, telling diabetics to, in effect, get half of their diet from sugar. They are concerned about the deadly plague of cardiovascular problems that people with diabetes face, and focusing on a low-fat diet as a result. Protein sends up a red flag to those worried about kidney disease, another common problem in diabetes. Carbs are basically what is left.

But it makes no sense whatsoever to feed carbs to people with what is basically a condition of carbohydrate intolerance. We know for sure that sugar (and the carbs it comes from) is not healthy for diabetics. And there's no evidence that otherwise healthy people who happen to have diabetes get kidney disease from eating protein, while heart problems have only been associated with certain kinds of fat (processed, saturated, or trans fats) that can simply be avoided. People with diabetes who keep their blood sugar levels normal avoid all these complications anyway.

Other experts, notably those at the American Institute for Cancer Research (AICR), have begun to develop more helpful guidelines placing emphasis on vegetables, fruit, whole grains, and beans—AICR wants them to cover at least two-thirds of your plate, for example. Scientists at the Harvard School of Public Health have developed their own "Healthy Eating Pyramid" focused on increased whole-grain foods, vegetables, and plant oils—and found that women adhering to it have 28 percent less heart disease than those following the standard pyramid from the USDA.

The pH Miracle plan takes their lead, moving away from carbohydrates and toward plant foods and healthy fats, but takes it even farther, so we can not just reduce risk, but (in many cases) eliminate it altogether. Why settle for less than glowing good health? Especially when you can attain it while feasting on nature's bounty?

THE pH MIRACLE PLAN FOR DIABETES

So here's your better way, in a nutshell: Cover your plate with vegetables. Seventy to 80 percent of your diet should come from fresh vegetables, grasses, sprouts, low-sugar fruits, and good fats (especially avocado and coconut). At least half of that should be raw. When you do cook, do so as quickly as possible, keeping your food to 118 degrees or less (you should be able to hold your finger in soup without having to pull it out immediately at that temperature), and add oils other than olive or grape seed to finished food, since they should never be heated.

The remaining 20 to 30 percent of your food should be fresh fish, nuts and seeds, and the grains that are only very mildly acidic: millet, buckwheat, and spelt. As long as you make wise choices, and limit it to no more than 20 percent of your diet, you might also decide to include some mildly acidic foods, perhaps some other grains or sweet or new potato.

Avoid processed foods, and choose organically grown food as much as possible to make sure your food reaches optimum nutrient levels, keeps all the nutrients it has, and isn't contaminated with the harsh chemicals of fertilizers and pesticides. Organic produce is as much as three times higher in nutrients than nonorganic.

Don't worry: Eating lots of raw vegetables doesn't mean you'll be living on iceberg topped with a wedge of orange-ish tomato. Shelley's recipes in chapter 10 will make all this easy—and delicious!—to implement. Our first book, *The pH Miracle,* provides a lot more details on how to eat this way, including getting the right equipment, learning some new food preparation techniques such as sprouting and dehydrating, food shopping, and keeping your pantry stocked. It contains a lot of other tempting recipes as well. That book also provides guidance on how to transition into this program. This isn't some fad diet, but a way of eating for a long and healthy lifetime, and taking your time in getting there makes it more likely you'll stay on the path you've chosen.

Chapter 8

Nutritional Supplements

*"Absorption and organization of sunlight,
the very essence of life on this planet, is almost
exclusively derived from plants. Plants are therefore
a biological accumulation of LIGHT. Since light is the
driving force of every cell in our bodies,
this is why we NEED PLANTS."*
—BIRCHER BENNER, M.D.

The standard American diet is "SAD" indeed, woefully insufficient in vitamins, minerals, and other critical nutrients, undernourishing your body while oversupplying it with calories and unhealthy fats. Even if you're one of the only 20 to 30 percent of Americans who actually meet the (decidedly minimal) goal of five servings of fruits or vegetables a day, you still might not get all you need for basic good health. Food quality has dropped considerably in the last few decades. Nutrients are destroyed by harvesting, storage, cooking, refrigeration, and reheating foods—not to mention the travesty of being processed until barely recognizable—and much of our food supply is grown in depleted soil that is deficient in or devoid of nutrients in the first place. Even following the pH Miracle plan, you can't count on getting everything you should out of your food. To nourish your body enough to reverse diabetes, you're going to need even more. You need a program of nutritional supplements designed specifically to make your body more alkaline. (Consult with your physician before beginning any nutritional supplement program.)

That's just what this chapter provides. Don't worry, it doesn't require handfuls of pills all day long. There's no one or two magic bullets either, though. But the basic recommendations for everyone are very reasonable: three supplements combined into one drink, plus two other types of supplements. Beyond that, there are two tiers of recommendations you can use to tailor a regimen to your specific situation. If you're eating right, a few careful selections will provide all you need to balance your body, stay alkaline, and put diabetes behind you. If you're *not* eating right, all the supplements in the world aren't going to bring you complete good health. The one–two punch of diet and supplements is the best way to prevent and reverse diabetes and live in total health.

FOUNDATION

With your daily green drinks, you're already getting three out of five of the most crucial supplements for preventing and reversing diabetes: green vegetable and grass powder, soy sprouts powder, and pH drops. More than a pound of produce is required to make just 1 ounce of **green powder,** and this incredible concentration means it is packed with vitamins and minerals, including those the pancreas most needs to protect and heal itself, along with chlorophyll, plant enzymes, and phytonutrients, as well as macronutrients like protein and fiber. By providing a rich source of alkaline substances (such as sodium, potassium, calcium, and magnesium) to maintain a healthy pH level in your body, green powder makes sure your body doesn't divert those minerals away from specific body systems (like the pancreas) that need them.

All the ingredients in the green powder you choose should be organically grown, then preserved through low-temperature dehydration. And of course you must mix it with the right water: distilled, purified, ionized—whatever you decide upon from the explanations about water in chapter 7.

Stir 1 teaspoon of green powder into 1 liter of water to make green drink, and get at least 3 to 4 liters per day.

GREEN POWDER

Look for many of these ingredients (which could also be taken as supplements) in whatever green powder you choose; all are useful in combating diabetes:

- Alfalfa juice concentrate
- Alfalfa leaf
- Aloe concentrate
- Barley grass
- Beta-carotene
- Bilberry leaf
- Black walnut leaf
- Blueberry leaf
- Boldo leaf
- Broccoli
- Cabbage
- Celery
- Cornsilk
- Couch grass
- Dandelion leaf
- Echinacea
- Goldenseal leaf
- Kale leaf
- Kamut grass
- Lecithin
- Lemongrass
- Marshmallow root
- Meadowsweet
- Oat grass
- Okra fruit
- Papaya leaf
- Parsley
- Pau d'arco root
- Pau d'arco root
- Plantain leaf
- Red raspberry leaf
- Rose hips
- Rosemary leaf
- Sage
- Shave grass
- Slippery elm bark
- Soy sprout
- Spearmint leaf
- Spinach
- Strawberry leaf
- Thyme
- Tomato
- Turmeric
- Watercress
- Wheatgrass
- White willow bark
- Wintergreen leaf

Soy sprouts powder is even more densely concentrated than the green powder, and rich in protein, enzymes, isoflavones, and other nutrients containing plant compounds that prevent and/or slow increasing or decreasing blood sugar levels and combat the acidity that can lead to diabetes. Isoflavones, already famous for helping lower cholesterol, inhibit atherosclerosis, prevent osteoporosis, and treat menopausal symptoms, are also a great support to the pancreas, and help balance blood sugar levels. The enzymes help prevent cellular damage and contain natural adaptogens, which help the body handle stress (stress that can lead to diabetes). Studies have demon-

VITAMINS AND MINERALS IN GREEN DRINK

The nutrients on this list, found in the vegetables and grasses in green powder and/or in soy sprouts powder, are all good for preventing or reversing diabetes. If you could find a multivitamin with all these things in it, it would be almost as potent as a green drink—though it would lack the power of chlorophyll.

• Alkaloids	• Germanium	• Phosphorous	• Thorium
• Aluminum	• Gold	• Platinum	• Thulium
• Antimony	• Hafnium	• Potassium	• Tin
• Arginine	• Holmium	• Praseodymium	• Titanium
• Barium	• Inosine	• Rhenium	• Tungsten
• Beryllium	• Iodine	• Rhodium	• Tyrosine
• Bismuth	• Iridium	• Rubidium	• Uranium
• Boron	• Iron	• Ruthenium	• Vanadyl
• Calcium	• Lanthanum	• Samarium	sulfate
• Cerium	• Lithium	• Scandium	• Vitamin A
• Cesium	• Lutetium	• Selenium	• Vitamin B_1
• Chromium	• Lysine	• Silicon	• Vitamin B_2
• Cobalt	• Magnesium	• Silver	• Vitamin B_6
• Copper	• Manganese	• Sodium	• Vitamin B_{12}
• Dysprosium	• Molybdenum	• Strontium	• Vitamin C
• Erbium	• Neodymium	• Sulfur	• Vitamin E
• Europium	• Nickel	• Tantalum	• Ytterbium
• Flavonoids	• Niobium	• Tellurium	• Yttrium
• Gadolinium	• Palladium	• Terbium	• Zinc
• Gallium	• Phenylalanine	• Thallium	• Zirconium

strated that soy is a natural way to balance hormone activity, ward off infection, detoxify the body, and even inhibit cancer-promoting agents. The soy plant contains unique protective compounds that counteract the process of fermentation as the body burns food for energy.

Add 1 scoop of soy sprout powder to each liter of green drink or water, or take 1 scoop directly by mouth three to four times per day.

Adding **pH drops** (what I call sodium chlorite and/or sodium silicate) to your green drinks (and plain water) increases the benefits of both the water and the green and soy sprout powders, making them still more alkalizing, oxygenating, and pH balancing. The pH drops act as oxygen and electron catalysts, bringing more of both into your blood and thus to all the cells of your body, which need it for optimum performance. The drops bind with chemicals in the water to release a highly active form of oxygen, making it easier for the body to absorb it, and helping stop negative transformations of microforms. They combine with sodium to make potassium, which is alkalizing.

Add 16 drops to each liter of water or green drink.

GREEN DRINK: GREEN POWDER, SOY SPROUTS POWDER, AND pH DROPS

The most powerful green drink contains 1 teaspoon of green powder, 1 scoop of soy sprouts powder, and 16 drops of pH drops. You should get at least 4 liters daily of green drinks—this will give you the benefits of more than 5 pounds of vegetables, grasses, and sprouts.

Drinking your vegetables (and grasses and sprouts) will help you regulate your blood sugar, neutralize acids, use glucose properly, prevent insulin resistance—in short, protect your body against the ravages of diabetes. This triple-threat combination completes three of the five bases all people facing diabetes need to cover in making the foundation of their supplement program. The fourth is an essential fatty acids (EFAs) supplement.

Essential fatty acids, as seen in chapter 7, help eliminate acids and protect against diabetes (and heart disease, stroke, high blood pressure, atherosclerosis, blood clots, and high cholesterol) and secondary symptoms of diabetes, including skin conditions, kidney dysfunction, and diabetic neuropathy. The omega-3 fatty acids EPA and DHA from fish have, in particular, been shown to prevent diabetes, as well as cardiovascular disease and stroke. In fact, a recent Italian study of more than eleven thousand people found that those who took 1 g of fish oil a day every day for three months reduced their risk of death from any health-related cause 41 percent compared to those taking a placebo. Fatty acids are essential to normal cell growth and maintenance. They are particular useful in the brain, eyes, and heart—among the most active tissues in the body. EFAs protect the insulin-producing beta cells of the pancreas from acid breakdown, and provide needed fats for building the membrane of every cell in the body.

ESSENTIAL FATTY ACIDS

I recommend a supplement combining fish and borage or hemp oils to properly balance omega-3s and omega-6s in a 3:1 ratio—the omega-3 fatty acids in fish oils (EPA and DHA) and omega-6's gamma-linolenic acid (GLA), linoleic acid (LA), and erucic acid (EA) in borage oil. You should take one 1,000 mg capsule three times a day. (In a serious condition—such as when you are beginning to deal with diabetes via the pH Miracle plan—you might temporarily take it six to nine times a day.)

Your fifth key supplement is a **broad-spectrum multivitamin and mineral supplement,** to make sure your body is receiving everything it needs each day to function properly. Look for one that includes mineral salts—what I like to call "cell salts"—which are ground into a fine powder for easy assimilation.

MULTI

The body can tolerate a deficiency of vitamins for longer than it can a deficiency of minerals—even a slight change in the blood concentration of important minerals can be life threatening. So be sure your multi provides both vitamins and minerals. Take a 500 mg capsule at least three times a day (six times a day when dealing with serious imbalances, including diabetes) with a green drink or water. Look for one containing all, or at least most, of the following, in approximately, but not necessarily precisely, the amounts listed:

Vitamins
- Vitamin A: 7,500 IU
- Vitamin B_1: 20 mg
- Vitamin B_2: 20 mg
- Vitamin B_6: 25 mg
- Vitamin B_{12}: 35 mcg
- Vitamin C: 350 mg
- Vitamin D: 150 IU
- Vitamin E: 300 IU
- Vitamin B_3 (niacinamide): 35 mg
- Biotin: 6 mg
- Choline: 150 mg

Minerals
- Calcium: 350 mg
- Magnesium: 350 mg
- Manganese: 200 mg
- Zinc: 10 mg
- Copper: 1 mg
- Potassium: 35 mg
- Selenium: 70 mcg
- Molybdenum: 40 mcg
- Silica: 10 mg

- Inositol: 15 mg
- Potassium iodine: 50 mcg

Mineral Salts

- Calcium phosphate (calc. phos.): 1 mg
- Ferric phosphate (ferr. phos.): 1 mg
- Potassium phosphate (kali. phos.): 1 mg
- Sodium phosphate (nat. phos.): 1 mg
- Sodium chloride (nat. mur.): 1 mg
- Sodium sulphate (nat. sulph.): 1 mg
- *Optional:* Calcium fluoride (calc. fluor.), calcium sulphate (calc. sulph.), potassium chloride (kali. mur.), potassium sulphate (kali. sulph.), magnesium phosphate (mag. phos.), and silica (si. oxide)

QUICK FIX FOR LOW BLOOD SUGAR

If you need to raise your blood sugar, don't resort to a big dose of sugar—which may do the job but also puts you directly into a very bad spiral. Instead, take 1 tablespoon soy sprouts powder with a liter of green drink with pH drops as a chaser, or mix the sprouts into the drink.

Mary Kay's Story

I was diagnosed with Type 2 diabetes in 1989, but if you can believe it, it was about the least of my health problems. I had congestive heart failure, early liver failure, and kidney failure. I had high blood pressure, a rapid heart rate, and mitral valve prolapse. I had an array of digestive problems, not least of which were bowel obstructions and the fact that 95 percent of my stomach lining was worn away. My eyesight was deteriorating, fluid was accumulating in my lungs, abdomen, feet, and ankles, and I needed to be hooked up to oxygen around the clock. I'd had at least a dozen surgeries, more than a hundred hospital stays, and an alarming array of medical diagnostic and treatment procedures, and took up to twelve different medications at a time.

Seven years later, I already had early signs of diabetic neuropathy, with pain in my legs and numbness and tingling in my feet. I struggled on this way for quite some time. By the beginning of this year, I was injecting two long-term and six short-term doses of insulin every day, on twenty-two units in the morning and five to ten at night.

Desperate, I started taking green drink with pH drops (in the small quantities my damaged stomach could handle). I also took supplements for heart, pancreas, kidney, and digestive system support, along with a multivitamin, and began eating an alkaline diet.

In just three days, my blood sugar dropped to within normal, nondiabetic range, and I started cutting my insulin doses. Within five weeks, I was off insulin altogether, and my blood sugars remained normal. A month later, I was off all but two of my medications, and off the oxygen. My blood pressure and heart rate normalized. My eyesight improved, and I had much more energy, and was even able to begin exercising. My stomach healed, and now I can eat green vegetables, legumes, nuts, and fruit without ending up in the hospital. And the doctors canceled the open-heart surgery they were prepping me for. The pH Miracle gave me my health back!

FRAMEWORK

With green drinks, EFAs, and a good multi, you've laid the foundation of your supplement program. For those who need or want to build up from there, I suggest some additional nutritional supplements, which I consider to be like the framework of a house. Not every house needs to be built with the exact same materials; what you use depends on the design you're following, which ideally would be suited specifically to you. Most people with diabetes would benefit from the supplements in this section. (There's no need to alter the recommended dose if anything that appears here is also found in your multivitamin.)

Chromium

Chromium, an essential mineral, increases the effectiveness of insulin, improving its ability to handle glucose. It stimulates the activity of enzymes involved in the metabolism of glucose for energy, and binds insulin and glucose together. By improving the uptake of sugar, chromium reduces acidity and so minimizes the body's need to retain fat. It also helps turn blood into muscle, and convert sugar into energy. Chromium is good for insulin resistance. Chromium inhibits the formation of plaque in your aorta, and deficiency can contribute to arterosclerosis. It also helps with weight loss.

Even a very slight deficiency in chromium will have serious effects on the body, upsetting the function of insulin, among other things, and thus leading to glucose intolerance. Although it is rare in other countries, deficiency is widespread in the United States. That's because our soil does not contain an adequate supply anymore, and thus chromium cannot be absorbed by crops or our water supply. Refining foods strips away much of any chromium that does manage to get there. Pregnant women are particularly susceptible to chromium deficiency because the fetus uses so much of it.

Animal studies dating back to 1957 showed that rats' tolerance of injected glucose was immediately restored in chromium-deficient rats when they received chromium supplements. More recent studies in people made the same point. In 1993, more than half of study participants with Type 2 diabetes, and more than a third of those with Type 1, were able to cut back on their oral hypoglycemic medication or insulin upon starting to take 200 mcg a day of chromium. In 1997, patients with Type 2 diabetes added chromium to their regimens without making any other changes in diet, medication, or activity level. When they had their blood sugar levels tested four months later, they had reductions in blood sugar and insulin, as well as cholesterol.

CHROMIUM

I've seen for myself what chromium can do for diabetics, or those with insulin sensitivities or glucose intolerance, especially in combination with the pH Miracle diet and exercise plan. I generally have my clients take 200 mcg of chromium three times a day, with a green drink or water. Most Americans fail to get even 50 mcg of chromium a day.

NADP

The natural coenzyme NADP reduces insulin resistance because it helps a form of glucose through the energy cycle of the cell. Without enough NADP in the body, you're at risk of insulin resistance and diabetes.

NADP (which, if you must know, stands for "B-nicotinamide adenine dinucleotide phosphate") is a cellular fuel for energy production; without it, no energy is produced. The more energy a cell needs, the more NADP it requires to obtain that energy. NADP helps retard cell death (including the pancreatic alpha and beta cells) and promotes tissue regeneration, as well as playing a key role in cell regulation and DNA repair. NADP is a potent anti-acid, and supports the white blood cells as they clear out negative microforms and their associated acids. NADP is good for the heart, too, lowering cholesterol and blood pressure. (NADP is present in every cell of the body, but the heart is particularly dense with it.)

NADH/P is a similar molecule found in humans; NADP is mainly found in plant sources. You might sometimes find co-Q1 or coenzyme Q1 in the store, which is basically the same thing.

NADP

Take 5 mg three times a day, on an empty stomach, with a green drink or a glass of water.

Vanadyl Sulfate

The essential trace mineral vanadyl sulfate helps control blood sugar. It mimics, in a key way, the action of insulin, stimulating the same transporters (known as "GLUT-4" transporters) for use in carrying glucose inside the cells. Numerous animal studies and a growing body of human research show that vanadyl sulfate improves fasting blood sugar levels. In a small study in 1996, for example, patients with Type 2 diabetes who took 50 mg of vanadyl sulfate twice a day for four weeks, and a placebo for four weeks, averaged a 20 percent drop in fasting blood sugar levels, a result so strong it even extended into the placebo period.

When combined with chromium, the duo helps control blood sugar levels as well as sugar cravings. They also lower LDL cholesterol and increase HDL cholesterol.

VANADYL SULFATE

I recommend taking 35 mg of vanadyl sulfate three times a day, with a green drink or water.

QUICK FIX FOR KETONES

• Superhydrate your body with a green drink with pH drops and NADP.
• Take chromium and vanadyl sulfate to bind insulin with glucose; just one dose works quickly.

Magnesium

Magnesium is involved in many essential metabolic processes. It activates enzymes necessary for the metabolism of carbohydrates (including sugar) and amino acids: You need sufficient magnesium in order to convert sugar into energy, preventing insulin resistance and excess acidity. Magnesium helps regulate the acid–alkaline balance in the blood and tissues. It is quite alkaline itself—in fact, it can be used in place of over-the-counter antacids. Magnesium also protects the heart and eyes, and helps the nerves function properly. Too little magnesium has been associated with heart disease, blood clot formation in the heart and brain, clogged arteries, high cholesterol, and diabetic retinopathy.

Magnesium deficiency is not uncommon, despite the fact that it appears in many foods, especially fresh green vegetables. But the mineral is refined out of many foods during processing, and cooking removes still more. And, of course, there are plenty of people who just don't eat their veggies. Several studies show that diabetic patients have below-average levels of magnesium in their blood, and higher losses of the mineral in their urine. Those put on magnesium supplements regain normal levels in their blood, and their risk of blindness and cardiovascular complications decreases.

Magnesium within the cell membrane is thought to enhance the effects of insulin. In a study of older people with Type 2 diabetes, participants taking 2 g of magnesium daily had significantly improved insulin sensitivity and glucose uptake compared to how they fared while taking a placebo.

MAGNESIUM

Magnesium should be balanced with manganese in a ratio of 2:1 when taken as a supplement. Take one 500 mg combination capsule three times a day with a green drink, water, or a meal. You might look for a supplement that includes herbs rich in magnesium: alfalfa, parsley, ginger, cayenne, gotu kola, yellow dock root, valerian root, and aloe vera extract.

Zinc

Your body needs zinc to make insulin, so this is obviously an important nutrient for diabetics. But people with diabetes are generally deficient in this essential trace mineral; their pancreases contain only about half as much zinc as those of healthy nondiabetics. Deficiencies may cause many pancreatic disorders (among many other things), including diabetes. It is worth noting, however, that too much zinc can be as harmful as too little; fortunately, there is a wide range between these two extremes where the body can make good use of zinc.

Zinc performs a variety of functions in the human body, including being involved in a number of metabolic processes. A constituent of at least twenty-five enzymes involved in digestion and metabolism, zinc is necessary for digesting carbs—including sugar—and is important in the normal absorption and action of most vitamins, especially those in the B complex. Zinc helps prevent or limit arteriosclerosis. In therapeutic doses, it speeds healing of wounds and injuries whether internal or external, including those related to diabetes. Zinc is a wonderful chelator, neutralizing acids foreign to the body. And it regulates insulin levels in the blood: Research shows that taking zinc along with insulin prolongs the effect of the insulin on blood sugar levels.

ZINC

Take a combination supplement containing at least 83 mg zinc amino acid chelate (a form of zinc combined with a protein) and 82 mg of zinc citrate three times a day (being sure not to get more than 1,800 mg a day of zinc). You might look for a supplement containing herbs rich in zinc, such as dandelion root, red clover, cayenne, echinacea leaf, parsley, gota kola, marshmallow root, chlorophyll, pumpkin seed lipids, and aloe vera extract.

Gymnema Sylvestre

The leaves of this climbing plant have been used in India for more than two thousand years to treat *madhu meha* ("honey urine")—what we call diabetes. It slows the absorption of sugars in the gastrointestinal tract, helps get sugar into the cells, and revitalizes insulin-producing beta cells in the pancreas.

In two studies, rats given toxic substances to induce diabetes and then given *Gymnema sylvestre* extracts for one to two months doubled the number of their beta cells and increased insulin levels to almost normal.

Human studies, too, have demonstrated gymnema's therapeutic value for both Type 1 and Type 2 diabetes. In one, people with Type 1 who took an extract for six to eight months reduced their average fasting blood sugar 23 percent, and cut their insulin doses by an average of 25 percent. In a study of people with Type 2, patients taking 400 mg a day of gymnema for eighteen to twenty months also had notable reductions in blood sugar—and all but one of the participants were able to significantly reduce their dosages of blood-sugar-lowering drugs. First of them managed to discontinue their medication altogether.

GYMNEMA SYLVESTRE

Take a 200 mg capsule three times a day with a green drink or water or with a meal. You'll need to work closely with your doctor to reduce the amount of insulin you take—if you are changing your diet at the same time, you'll see a change within three days that could necessitate a drop by as much as half of your insulin dose. Check your blood sugar levels at least three times a day.

Fenugreek

Fenugreek seeds have been shown, in lab research on animals, to decrease blood sugar levels, as well as total cholesterol and tri-glycerides.

FENUGREEK

Take one 500 mg capsule of fenugreek seeds three times a day.

Bitter Melon

Bitter melon, also known as balsam pear or bitter gourd, is a tropical fruit, available in this country mainly as an extract, sold as a supplement. It can reduce blood sugar levels, including in Type 1 diabetics, by increasing the cells' uptake of sugar.

One study showed that people with Type 2 who took 15 g of bitter melon extract after a meal for three weeks cut their blood sugars in half. After seven weeks, 73 percent of the group had a significant lowering of blood sugar, putting them in the normal-high range for a nondiabetic.

Bitter melon also alkalinizes the whole body, reducing systemic acids.

BITTER MELON

Take 3 to 4 ounces of bitter melon juice in 1 liter or quart of distilled water at least once a day, or anytime you need to reduce high blood sugar levels.

Clay

For those of you who don't think I've gone far enough in telling you to subsist mainly on plants, I'm going to up the ante by also recommending you eat dirt.

You heard right: dirt. But not just any dirt. The dirt I recommend is Montmorillonite clay, from its namesake deposit near Montmorillon, France, where it was first identified. Hang in there; this will make more sense once you know what clay contains, what it does for the body, and how you use it.

Clay provides an impressive assortment of minerals, including calcium, iron, magnesium, potassium, manganese, sodium, and silica, all of which are alkalinizing. What's more, in clay the minerals exist in natural proportion to one another, so they are more easily and thoroughly absorbed by the body. The clay carries a negative electric charge, so it attracts toxins and acids from fermenting sugar, which are positively charged, and holds them in suspension so the body can safely eliminate the whole package. It can do this to toxins even many times its own weight.

Clay improves a long list of ailments and illnesses, not least being diabetes. I've had clients report reducing their use of insulin and even getting off it altogether. Others told me their sugar levels balanced out, or they lost weight. You should notice a difference within two to four weeks of starting to take clay.

Montmorillonite clay is all natural, with no additives, chemicals, or preservatives. The only processing it undergoes is crushing. And while it might not be the most delicious thing in the pH Miracle plan, it doesn't really taste bad—a little salty, though. You can buy Montmorillonite clay in health food stores (just be sure not to confuse it with the less active but more widely available bentonite clay from Wyoming), or through our Web site (see the resources section).

CLAY

I recommend 6 to 8 ounces of clay mixtures, two or three times a day. There are a number of ways you can use Montmorillonite clay, and you may want to try different ones to find which you like best:

- Mix 1 teaspoon of dry powder Montmorillonite clay in a half glass of distilled water and let it sit for six to eight hours (don't leave a metal spoon in it). Either drink the clear liquid off the top, or stir it up and drink the whole thing. Some people get better results taking it first thing in the morning, some prefer to take it the last thing at night, and some do best at different times during the day. Again, you'll have to experiment.

- Stir 1 heaping tablespoon of Montmorillonite clay "mixed gel" into half a glass of water or green drink and take immediately. Some people find the gel has less of a noticeable taste to it.

- You can use the clay externally, too, where it is good for a number of ailments from bee stings and mosquito bites to diaper rash and boils. Of most importance to someone with diabetes would be clay's ability to help heal sores. Make a paste the consistency of mustard by mixing water and clay gel in roughly a 2:1 ratio. Apply directly to the skin, uncovered if you want a tightening effect, or covered if you want a more cooling and soothing effect. Apply once or twice daily; you can leave it on overnight if desired. Just rinse it off with water and gentle rubbing when you are done. You can also simply sprinkle clay powder directly on a wound.

SUPPLEMENTS FOR THE LIQUID FEAST

Our first book, *The pH Miracle,* provides more details about the following supplements for use during a liquid feast. You will benefit from a liquid feast without them, but using them will give you the most efficient and effective results.

Herbal Cleanser

During your initial liquid feast, I recommend a special blend of supplements to provide a balanced source of daily fiber. Choose one designed to cleanse your body—bowels, liver, kidney, lungs, skin, and pancreas—from years of overacidity. Look for an all-natural synergistic combination of herbs that should include many if not all of the following: **butternut root bark, cascara sagrada bark, turkey rhubarb root, psyllium seeds,** and **Irish moss** for their laxative properties; **ginger** and **licorice roots** for their ability to ease discomfort in the colon, restore tone, and heal membranes; and **cayenne, barberry root, fennel seed oil,** and **red raspberry leaves** for the various ways they improve digestion. Other beneficial ingredients include **wheat bran, alfalfa, parsley,** and **apple pectin.** This combination provides plenty of fiber to help the digestive system eliminate waste, both by improving intestinal mobility and by binding with acids to remove them from the gut.

Take supplement with water or a green drink during the liquid feast as follows:

- Adults over 60: One or two 500 mg capsules every eight hours.
- Adults 22–60: Four 500 mg capsules every four hours.
- Ages 16–21: Two or three 500 mg capsules every six hours.
- Ages 6–16: Two or three 500 mg capsules every eight hours.
- Ages 5 and under: Not recommended. You can use bulk laxatives, such as psyllium seed by itself.

You might also want to use **aloe vera** during your liquid feast, to break up protein in the intestine and help in healing structures within the intestine. Besides its cleansing power, aloe vera contains vitamins, minerals, amino acids, enzymes, and lipids. It has also been shown to lower blood sugar levels in people with Type 2 diabetes—in one study, enough to allow participants to cut their dose of oral medication in half while maintaining normal blood sugar levels. Take 1 tablespoon of whole leaf aloe vera juice six to nine times daily during the liquid feast. (Beyond the liquid feast, aloe vera is good for anyone with continuing lower-bowel issues; take 1 tablespoon three times a day on an empty stomach—upon waking, before lunch, and before going to bed.)

Liquid Supplements

You should be able to find liquid colloidal forms of these supplements at your local health food store. Although I've listed all the ingredients separately, you should be able to get combined formulas to keep down the number of bottles you have to deal with.

Take 5 drops under the tongue of these liquid colloidal supplements, one after the other:

- B complex
- Caprylic
- Iridium
- Magnesium
- Manganese
- N-acetyl cysteine
- NADH
- Noni (no sugar, not fermented or pasteurized)
- Rhodium
- Silver

- Trace minerals (from a broad-spectrum mineral-based supplement)
- Undecylenic

Capsule Supplements

Once again, look for combination formulas to reduce the number of pills you need.

- Lower-bowel-cleansing formula (for severe bowel congestion, a more intense formula than the herbal cleanser above, with a higher concentration of cascara sagrada): Four 500 mg capsules if you're under sixty-five, two 500 mg capsules if you're sixty-six or older.
- Formula including caprylic and undecylenic, to fight yeast: One 500 mg capsule.
- Formula including n-acetyl cysteine, to fight acid: One 500 mg capsule.
- Noni formula: One 500 mg capsule.
- Multivitamin: One 500 mg capsule.
- Magnesium/manganese formula: One 500 mg capsule.
- Zinc formula: One 500 mg capsule.

Finally, for any specific health challenges you are struggling with, you should add a capsule of the relevant support formula. Besides those described in the Roof section, diabetics might find particularly useful formulas designed to help the kidneys, lungs, or reproductive system (male or female), or to help with allergies, inflammation, or mood.

ROOF

Now you're ready for the finishing touches to your program of supplements. If you were building a house, this would be the roof. The building will stand without a roof, but one is highly recommended for ultimate success!

Many of the supplements in this section are aimed at people with specific health challenges beyond diabetes. If you have diabetes, high blood pressure, and adrenal stress, for example, you should take the supplements that support the pancreas, heart, and adrenal glands. If you are having thyroid problems in addition to sugar imbalances, you should use the thyroid support supplement.

In any case, look for synergistic formulas designed to support diabetes to give you many vitamins, minerals, and herbs in combination, in the interest of limiting the number of capsules you need to take.

Glandulars

I recommend using glandulars—nucleic acid compounds isolated from defatted, dehydrated animal organs—in combination with other nutrients to balance and support the various glandular organs of the body. Studies show that glandulars can make up for deficiencies by delivering nutrients to the same organ in your body that they originate from in an animal. For example, bovine pancreas will bring nucleic acids directly to the pancreas. Raising the level of nucleic acids in an organ renews its ability to function well. Look for "bovine pancreas" or "bovine heart" on the label, to give just two examples.

Vitamin E

Your multi will surely include vitamin E, but you may want to include additional amounts in your routine. Vitamin E inhibits the formation of acid when you eat protein, and chelates acids so your body can get rid of them. It builds immunity and strengthens your body's defense against environmental toxins. Vitamin E helps counter the gradual decline in metabolic process that comes with aging—not only effectively slowing aging, but also helping prevent unwanted weight gain (the dreaded "middle-age spread"). In lab studies, animals given vitamin E lived longer than those who weren't.

Vitamin E comes with a long list of conditions it benefits, but of most interest to diabetics is its ability to improve insulin sensitivity. And Dr. Evan Shute reports that fully a quarter of his diabetic patients decreased how much insulin they needed by ten or more units by taking vitamin E every day. Vitamin E protects against chronically elevated blood sugar levels, and it can clear up or control many forms of kidney disease, protect your eyes, keep your skin healthy, and prevent gangrene.

Perhaps most important of all, to diabetics and everyone else, is the way vitamin E protects against heart disease. It improves circulation, the supply of blood to the heart, and hemoglobin's ability to carry oxygen. It reduces clotting as well as dissolving scars on arterial walls that can otherwise cause blockages, and binding to and neutralizing acids on artery walls. Vitamin E helps the heart use oxygen more efficiently. When you remember that heart attacks can be caused by clots and/or low oxygen levels to the heart, you can see how important vitamin E can be. In a study of more than two thousand patients, one group took between 400 and 800 IUs of vitamin E a day, while the other took a pill of inactive ingredients as a placebo. They were followed for nearly a year and a half. During that time, those taking the supplement had 75 percent fewer heart attacks.

Besides preventing heart attacks, vitamin E is a boon even when heart attacks do occur: Looking again at Dr. Shute's work, he reports that heart attack patients with sufficient levels of vitamin E are more likely to survive the attack, and will sustain less tissue damage. Vitamin E helps prevent angina and lower cholesterol levels. By reducing acid throughout your body, it also helps prevent fat deposits.

You get vitamin E—tocopherols—in high concentrations in cold-pressed vegetable oils, whole raw seeds and nuts, and soybeans. Beyond what you get in food, I recommend a special formulation of vitamin E that is natural, dry, and virtually oil-free, in a chewable tablet, ideally combined with chromium and selenium for added effectiveness. Dried vitamin E is better absorbed than traditional oil-encapsulated vitamin E. Look for the "alpha-tocopherols" form of vitamin E, which is the most potent. Take 200 IUs three times a day.

B Vitamins

This is another case where you might want to do a little better than your basic multi, particularly for vitamins B_1 (thiamine), B_3 (niacin), and B_6. The B vitamins act to convert carbohydrates into glucose for the body to burn for energy, and are vital in the metabolism of fats and proteins as well. Of particular interest to people with diabetes, B vitamins are also essential for normal functioning of the nervous system—they are perhaps the single most important factor in health of the nerves—as well as being important to the health of the heart, skin, eyes, and mouth, among much else. (The use of birth control pills can cause deficiencies of B vitamins, so anyone taking them should consider supplementation.)

Among the benefits of **vitamin B_1** are that it stabilizes the appetite and improves food digestion and absorption, particularly of starches and sugars. A deficiency makes it difficult to digest carbohydrates, leading to too much sugar in the blood. People with diabetes should note that thiamine deficiency can also lead to inflammation of the optic nerve, central nervous system dysfunction, and heart irregularities and cardiac damage. Mild deficiency is hard to detect and is often attributed to other problems; the signs include fatiguing easily, loss of appetite, irritability, and emotional instability. Moderate deficiency can cause digestive and memory problems.

And many Americans are deficient in vitamin B_1. The main reason is that it is processed out of foods during refining or cooking, or even just exposure to air or water.

Vitamin B_3 comes in two forms, niacin and nicotinamide. **Nicotinamide** may preserve and/or improve the functioning of beta cells in the pancreas. It has even served to actually reverse Type 1 diabetes in some patients when administered properly within the first few years of diagnosis. (Follow recommendations below as soon as you know you have an issue.) In a large study in New Zealand, more than twenty thousand five- to seven-year-olds were screened for islet cell antibodies (ICA), indicating a high risk of developing Type 1 diabetes. Most of the high-risk children identified agreed to take the offered nicotinamide therapy, and those who did showed a 60 percent decrease in the rate of diabetes over the seven years (on average) they were followed.

Niacin has also been useful in patients who are at high risk of developing Type 1 diabetes. In addition, it has been shown to assist in weight reduction in people with Type 2 diabetes, thanks to its ability to stabilize blood sugar levels. That same trick makes it helpful for hypoglycemia as well. Furthermore, niacin improves circulation, reduces cholesterol levels, and helps keep the digestive and nervous systems healthy, as well as the skin and the tongue.

I recommend both forms, although you should be aware of the "niacin rush" that sometimes accompanies that form. It's a good sign, actually—increased circulation—but some people find it unpleasant.

Take 100 mg of each three times a day; you might want to begin with 25 mg of each and work up from there if you want to avoid the rush reaction.

Vitamin B$_6$ (pyridoxine) deficiency results in low blood sugar, low glucose tolerance, and insulin insensitivity. It can also look like some side effects of diabetes, causing nerve disorders, increased urination, and visual disturbances. Vitamin B$_6$ is needed for proper digestion of food, including the breakdown and utilization of carbohydrates and sugars. It also facilitates the release of stored glycogen (sugar) from the liver and muscles for energy. And B$_6$ helps maintain the ratio between sodium and potassium that is critical to the body's delicate pH balance.

Diabetics tend to have lower levels of B$_6$ than healthy people. An Australian study of five hundred people with diabetes proved not only that point, but also that diabetics with cardiovascular problems had even lower levels of the vitamin than diabetics in general. Not unrelated is the fact that B$_6$ assists in cholesterol metabolism and the control of arteriosclerosis. In other good news for diabetics in particular, B$_6$ can be used in treating nervous disorders, elevated cholesterol, and some heart disturbances, tooth problems, and skin problems. It is also a powerful antacid.

B_6 supplementation has been shown to be a safe treatment for gestational diabetes; one clinical trial reported in the *British Medical Journal* showed that pregnant women taking 100 mg daily of B_6 for just two weeks experienced complete reversal of their diabetes.

Vitamin B_{12} can reduce nerve damage caused by diabetes. A 1995 study in *Current Therapeutic Research* found that nerve pain, and nerve damage due to diabetes, were significantly reduced, and nerve function significantly improved, in participants who took supplemental B_{12}.

I recommend taking a 500 mg B-complex capsule three times a day, with a green drink, water, or a meal. My favorite is combined with a blend of herbs including skullcap, gingerroot, hops, valerian root, and cayenne, with roughly the following amounts of the various B vitamins:

- Vitamin B_1: 50 mg
- Vitamin B_2: 50 mg
- Vitamin B_3: 50 mg
- Vitamin B_4 or choline bitartrate: 50 mg
- Vitamin B_5 or pantothenic acid: 50 mg
- Vitamin B_6: 50 mg
- Vitamin B_7 or biotin: 100 mcg
- Vitamin B_8 or inositol: 50 mg
- Vitamin B_9 or folic acid: 400 mcg
- PABA: 25 mg
- Vitamin B_{12}: 500 mcg

Pancreatic Support Supplement

I often recommend to my clients a blend of herbs, combined with micronutrients, chromium, cell salts, amino acids, and fatty acids, to promote healthy pancreatic functioning. Glandulars in the mix provide nucleic acids that collect and deliver the other nutrients directly to the pancreas. The herbs cleanse, detoxify, and invigorate the pancreas, as well as stimulating circulation, improving digestion and strengthening other glands and organs, including the kidneys, among a host of other benefits. Used regularly, together with green drink and green foods, the effect of these herbs can be extraordinary, giving you a vital pancreas (and much more) for life. As a supplement to insulin therapy, this mix supports all the physiological systems involved to the point that it ameliorates prediabetic and diabetic conditions in many individuals, including lessening the need for insulin. The primary active herbal ingredients you should look for follow. They all have a spectrum of beneficial properties, but here I'll mention only the ones of particular interest to people with diabetes:

- *Uva-ursi* helps protect the pancreas, kidneys, and many glands, and helps lower blood sugar.
- *Dandelion root* seems to lower or stabilize blood sugar (though more research is needed to determine just how that happens) and is generally good for the health of the pancreas.
- *Parsley* is an antacid and helps lower blood sugar levels.
- *Gentian root* works primarily in the digestive system (including the pancreas), affecting appetite, digestion, and absorption of nutrients. It also has antacid properties. Gentian root has secondary effects on other organs, such as the kidneys. Gentian root helps lower blood sugar, and may delay the onset of—or entirely prevent—"brittle" diabetes (with unpredictable spikes and dives in blood sugar levels).
- *Raspberry leaf* lowers blood sugar levels, as well as relieving urinary tract and kidney irritation.
- *Huckleberry leaf* contains similar blood-sugar-lowering compounds as its close cousin uva-ursi. This is one of the best herbs for people with mild diabetes, and is especially beneficial for those with "senile" diabetes—diabetes occurring with increasing age (usually in the sixties or seventies), complicated by degeneration of other parts of the body.
- *Buchu leaf* also relieves irritation of the bladder and kidneys.
- *Saw palmetto berry* helps build new tissue and restore function, including in the systems involved in diabetes.
- *Kelp* is useful primarily for its iodine, which it absorbs from seawater. Kelp also sponges up a variety of other essential

nutrients, including EFAs, trace elements, and sodium and potassium salts; it contains biologically important amounts of iron, copper, magnesium, calcium, potassium, barium, boron, chromium, lithium, nickel, silica, silver, stronidium, titanium, vanadyl sulfate, and zinc. Kelp's iodine is crucial for proper regulation of metabolism, helping the body burn off excess sugar and avoiding the buildup of fat that comes from binding up acids created from sugar metabolism. Kelp is an antacid.

- *Bladder wrack*—another sea weed—helps with obesity, heart damage and disease, and some kidney problems.

Other herbs that support the pancreas include **licorice root, alfalfa, blue vervain, aloe vera, Siberian ginseng, cedar berries,** and **blue cohosh.** Look for a variety of all these herbs, in combination with the following vitamins and minerals:

- Vitamin A: 2,000 IU
- B_1: 0.7 mg
- B_2: 0.75 mg
- B_3: 5 mg
- Vitamin E: 13.5 IU
- Pantothenic acid: 6.4 mg
- Zinc amino acid chelate: 0.9 mg
- Magnesium amino acid chelate: 35 mg
- Manganese amino acid chelate: 10 mg
- Chromium amino acid chelate: 0.25 mg
- Selenium amino acid chelate: 0.01 mg
- Calcium phosphate: 1 mg
- Potassium chloride: 1 mg
- Potassium sulphate: 1 mg
- Magnesium phosphate: 1 mg
- Sodium phosphate: 1 mg
- Silica: 1 mg

Take one 500 mg capsule six times a day with a green drink, water, or a meal. It is fine to take this along with a multi, and B and E supplements.

Allison's Story

I've been on insulin for twenty-three years, up to 120 units a day, plus two oral medications besides. Nothing ever helped. Still my blood sugars were out of control, usually over 400, sometimes closer to 500. I had polyneuropathy of my right foot—not much feeling in it—and the feeling in my left foot was almost entirely gone. Every time I walked into a doctor's office, I was told to lose weight—and add ten units of insulin.

Besides diabetes, I was a walking encyclopedia of poor health, taking multiple medications and living with constant pain. I had no energy, could barely walk. I had to quit even going shopping, and I was afraid to take care of my grandchildren on my own. I've worked in the health care field for over thirty years now, and was skeptical that anything would work for me. I hit my low point in my midfifties, when I was diagnosed with cirrhosis of the liver and told I had six months to two years to live.

That was four years ago.

After I got really, really sick, I found the pH Miracle program for controlling diabetes and started taking green drink with pH drops. I also began on pancreas and adrenal support supplements, EFAs, chromium, vanadium, NADH, and a multivitamin with cell salts. In four weeks, I lost 18 pounds, and in three months I was off my insulin injections!

By now I'm up to 4 liters of green drink a day, and I've shed 73 pounds, and counting. I'm still taking oral medications, but only two rather than three times a day. I'm starting to have *low* blood sugar throughout the day, so I'm cutting even that in half now. My goal is to get off medication completely, and I don't think it will take too much longer. (I'm already off all my other meds.) My blood sugars run consistently below 160 now.

I was so obese I couldn't exercise, but now I've started walking more. I park in the farthest parking lot at the hospital where I work to get at least two little walks a day, coming and going. I move easily and without pain. The feeling in my feet is back, with the exception of just one of my big toes.

I've changed my diet now, too, and try to keep it alkaline. When I get off track, my body lets me know! I begin to ache, my muscles are stiff, and I retain fluid in reaction to the acid I put into my body. (Not to mention the fat my body adds to protect itself.)

I still would like to lose about 150 more pounds, and for the first time in my life I feel I am really going to do it. It has always been such a chore to lose weight, and I've always put it all back on, plus a few more, in just a few months. But this plan is not a chore. I feel so much better, and have an enormous amount of energy. I can go, go, go.

The pH Miracle saved my life. I am feeling like living again. And I'm back to feeling able to take care of my seven wonderful grandchildren myself sometimes. Last Christmas I kept all of them while my kids did some last-minute shopping. They are the joy of my life, and I plan to be around to see them grow up!

Adrenal Support Supplement

Your adrenal glands create and release crucial hormones, and are famous for orchestrating that "adrenaline rush" that equips you to take action in emergencies. In real life, however, you call on your adrenals to cope with stress more often than with true emergencies. But because we are under such constant stress from so many sources (physical, emotional, and psychological, including but certainly not limited to the stresses of inadequate diet, exercise, exposure to external toxins, excess bodily acidity, and chronic illness), we force our adrenal glands into overdrive and, eventually, exhaustion. Their activity gradually decreases, and they may ultimately fail completely.

Adrenal glands also speed metabolism and improve circulation, and both systems suffer when you are subject to too much stress.

The adrenal glands increase red blood cell count, delivering more oxygen to the cells so they can burn fuel faster, and also increase the supply of fuel by stimulating the liver and muscles to release sugar into the bloodstream. Your adrenal glands, that is, provide you with energy. But on the flip side, this means that when too much stress leads to too much adrenal action, you'll be on the path to high blood sugar, then high insulin levels and insulin resistance—then alpha and beta cell burnout and eventually diabetes.

You should give your adrenals a break by reducing the stress you are under as much as you can. Learn to relax. Take good care of yourself. But living in this modern world means living with stress— and diabetes itself is extremely stressful, and continually activates the adrenals—so you need to keep your adrenals functioning in top form to help you handle it as gracefully as possible. You can support your adrenals using a combination of vitamins, minerals, herbs, cell salts, and glandulars to give your adrenal system all the necessary materials to keep itself in good repair, minimizing the damaging effects of daily stress.

Adrenal glandular is a key component of that combination. It provides all the nutrients necessary to support the human adrenal system, and takes them directly to the adrenals. The other crucial ingredient is **pantothenic acid** (vitamin B_5), commonly in the form of d-calcium pantothenate. Pantothenic acid is dramatically decreased in most foods during processing, cooking, freezing, and/or thawing. In your body, levels tend to decline with age, which comes with an accompanying decrease in ability to withstand stress. Animal studies show that in rats fed a diet devoid of pantothenic acid, the adrenal glands were destroyed. Studies on humans (modeled after studies of rats) show that very high doses (up to a thousand times the U.S. recommended daily allowance) daily for six weeks prevented almost all physiological stress-related problems and bodily damage resulting from a swim in water below 50 degrees Fahrenheit.

I recommend an adrenal support combination that includes some or all of these beneficial herbs: licorice root, alfalfa, parsley, chickweed, juniper berries, saw palmetto berries, cayenne, echinacea leaf, and Mexican saffron. Finally, look for something with nutrient levels roughly equivalent to these:

- Vitamin B_2: 0.76 mg
- Vitamin B_3: 9.0 mg
- Vitamin B_5: 100.0 mg
- Vitamin B_6: 0.9 mg
- Glandular adrenals: 25 mg
- Iodine: 60 mcg
- Calcium phosphate: 1 mg
- Calcium sulphate: 1 mg
- Potassium phosphate: 1 mg
- Potassium sulphate: 1 mg

To help *prevent* symptoms of adrenal stress, take one 500 mg capsule three times a day with green drink, water, or a meal. To help *reduce* the symptoms of adrenal stress, take it six times a day.

QUICK FIX FOR OVERACIDITY

To get rid of acid quickly:

- Take 1,000 mg each of pancreas and adrenal support supplements.
- Take chromium and vanadyl sulfate together, preferably in liquid form.

Thyroid Support Supplement

Many of the side effects of diabetes can be traced to an underactive thyroid gland: weight gain, obesity, poor teeth, elevated cholesterol, heart problems, fatigue, and much more. The thyroid gland regulates the rate of metabolism and how much energy the body burns. A healthy, active thyroid produces hormones that are vital to maintaining normal metabolism. The main thyroid hormones stimulate the activity of many organs, including the pancreas, tissues, and cells.

The thyroid works closely with the pancreas and the adrenal glands in regulating the body's energy needs, and stress on one will quickly throw the others off. When the pancreas is not functioning correctly, the thyroid gland will in all likelihood be overstressed, nutritionally depleted, and underactive as well—and vice versa. So for many people, supplementing to support the thyroid is a good idea. There are several herbs that can help, and following is a list of beneficial ones to look for in a combination capsule:

- *Kelp* is the key ingredient in any supplement targeting the thyroid gland, because of the iodine it supplies. The thyroid gland is the body's main repository of iodine, and requires the intake of iodine for proper development and functioning, including production of its main hormone.
- *Gentian root* helps normalize the thyroid, if indirectly.
- *Cayenne* stimulates glandular activity and provides important vitamins and minerals.
- *Irish moss,* a close relative of kelp, also supplies iodine (and other electrolyte minerals including calcium, magnesium, and sodium), trace elements, and tissue salts. It enhances the detoxifying functions of the digestive system, and increases the metabolic rate.

Other beneficial herbs include dulse, goldenrod, guarana root, wheatgrass, and barley grass. Look for a variety of the above in combination with the following nutrients, in roughly the recommended amounts:

- Vitamin C: 27 mg
- Vitamin E: 10.5 IU
- Iodine (kelp): 300 mcg
- Calcium amino acid chelate: 40 mg
- Iron amino acid chelate: 20 mg
- Micro bovine pituitary complex: 10 mg
- Micro bovine thyroid complex: 10 mg
- Calcium sulphate: 1 mg
- Sodium chloride: 1 mg

- Potassium chloride: 1 mg
- Potassium sulphate: 1 mg

Take one 500 mg capsule at least three times a day, with a green drink, water, or a meal.

Heart Health Supplement

For those struggling with or concerned about heart health—and all diabetics fall into one or the other of those groups—I recommend a blend of herbs to protect the heart:

- *Hawthorn berry* should be the "heart" of any such combination; it boasts more than a century of effectiveness against various faces of cardiovascular disease. Lab work and clinical studies in this country and around the world have shown that hawthorn berry boosts blood flow to the heart, improves circulation, lowers blood pressure, increases enzyme metabolism in the heart muscle (increasing energy), normalizes heartbeat, rhythm, rate, and pulse, and improves efficiency of oxygen use in the heart. It can be helpful in treating angina and atherosclerosis. (It is worth noting that hawthorn berry appears to work in synergy with digitalis, and using them together may well dramatically decrease the amount of digitalis required.) With all these benefits—and a solid reputation for being essentially free of negative side effects—it is easy to understand why hawthorn berry is so widely used in other countries. What's puzzling is why it has not received much attention in mainstream medical circles in the United States.
- *Cayenne,* acting as a stimulant, assures delivery of the other active ingredients in this blend, and helps activate them. In addition, it contains important nutrients for the health of the circulatory system. Cayenne and hawthorn berry taken together augment each other, so you should look for the pairing.
- *Motherwort,* also known, subtly enough, as heart wort, heart gold, heart heal, or heart herb, is used all over the world as a

cardiac tonic. It lowers blood pressure, prevents spasms of the blood vessels, and is calming, acting as a relaxant. Motherwort normalizes heart function in general—calming palpitations, for instance. And it is good for circulation. Motherwort is at its best when it can work in conjunction with other herbs with similar activity.

- *Rosemary leaf* is rich in minerals such as calcium, magnesium, phosphorus, sodium, and potassium that the heart (not to mention nerves) needs to function properly. Like motherwort, rosemary leaf works best in combination with like herbs.
- *Kelp* reduces acid, lowers blood pressure, and provides crucial nutrients, all of which enhance the effectiveness of the herbal blend.

Other good ingredients to look out for include buckwheat flour, black cohosh, rutin, peppermint, licorice root, acerola, gentian root, garlic, red beet root, skullcap, parsley, watercress, and *Allium sativa*. In addition, to provide nutritional support to the heart, look for the vitamins, minerals, glandulars, and cell salts in approximately the amounts given below:

- Vitamin A: 2000 IU
- Vitamin B_1: 10 mg
- Vitamin B_2: 3 mg
- Vitamin B_3: 4.5 mg
- Vitamin B_6: 5 mg
- Vitamin B_{12}: 0.05 mg
- Vitamin D: 50 IU
- Vitamin E: 400 IU
- Pantothenic acid: 15 mg
- Folic acid: 0.02 mg
- Biotin: 0.01 mg
- Choline: 50 mg
- Inositol: 8 mg
- PABA: 5 mg
- Calcium amino acid chelate: 30 mg
- Iron amino acid chelate: 20 mg

- Magnesium amino acid chelate: 30 mg
- Manganese amino acid chelate: 10 mg
- Zinc amino acid chelate: 10 mg
- Potassium amino acid chelate: 5 mg
- Selenium amino acid chelate: 2 mg
- Copper amino acid chelate: 0.06 mg
- Chromium amino acid chelate: 0.02 mg
- Whole bovine adrenal: 10 mg
- Whole bovine spleen: 10 mg
- Whole bovine thymus: 10 mg
- Micro bovine arterial tissue complex: 10 mg
- Calcium phosphate: 1 mg
- Magnesium phosphate: 1 mg
- Ferric phosphate: 1 mg
- Potassium phosphate: 1 mg
- Silica: 1 mg

Take one 500 mg capsule at least three times a day with a green drink, water, or a meal.

Liver Formulation

The combination of herbs given here benefits all the filter organs, the liver prime among them, but also the kidneys, lungs, and skin. They cleanse, purify, and detoxify those organs and the blood. Use them anytime you need to detoxify from overacidity, or to support the body during recuperation from any harmful condition (diabetes, for example). This will work especially well in combination with essential fatty acids, soy sprouts, and the pancreas support formula.

- *Dandelion* helps the body eliminate acids and negative micro-forms.
- *Red clover* alone helps detox and purify the blood and the organs (like the liver) that filter it; combine it with **kelp, stillingia,** and **burdock root,** and you'll have a most powerful blood cleanser.

- *Buckthorn and cascara sagrada bark* influence the gastrointestinal tract.
- *Licorice root, burdock root, and sarsaparilla root* generally strengthen and tone the liver, and have stimulating properties as well.
- *Chaparral, Oregon grape root, and prickly ash* benefit the glands in the mucous membranes, reducing acidity, thus reducing the production of mucus necessary to bind to acid as a protective mechanism, and support an impressive array of vital physiological and metabolic activities.

You should also look for glandular liver (bovine), yellow dock root, celery seed, echinacea, cayenne, wild yam root, barberry bark, red beet root, parsley, and hops. In addition, you should get a formula that includes the following vitamins, minerals, and cell salts in approximately the doses given:

- Vitamin B_3: 3 mg
- Vitamin B_6: 0.3 mg
- Vitamin B_{12}: 0.0006 mg
- Pantothenic acid: 2 mg
- Calcium: 500 mg
- Iodine: 0.0225 mg
- Zinc amino acid chelate: 5.5 mg
- Magnesium amino acid chelate: 4 mg
- Potassium chloride: 2 mg
- Calcium sulphate: 2 mg
- Magnesium phosphate: 2 mg
- Sodium sulphate: 2 mg
- Silica: 2 mg

Take one 1,000 mg capsule six to nine times a day with a green drink, water, or a meal.

HERBS FOR DIABETES
AND RELATED SYMPTOMS

These can be included in a green drink, used as part of a combination capsule, or taken on their own, following package directions. Essentially all the symptoms listed here are due to excessive acid production within the body; these herbs in general fight overacidity. To determine which herbs would be most helpful in your particular case, choose those that address your specific symptoms, and look for some or all of them in a combination capsule. The exact amounts are less important than getting the right herbs.

HERBAL OVERVIEW	
Herb	*Benefit*
Bilberry leaves	Helps improve blood sugar control in diabetics, lowers triglycerides, strengthens capillaries, protects against atherosclerosis, and blocks *E. coli* bacteria.
Boldo	Treats indigestion, protects the liver from metabolic acids, has anti-inflammatory and antimicrobial properties.
Goldenseal	Has antifungal and antibacterial properties and helps neutralize system acids in the gut, blood, and tissues.
Lecithin	May lower cholesterol, may protect liver against sugar-produced acids.
White willow	Anti-inflammatory, anti-acid.
Slippery elm	Treats irritable bowel syndrome, gastritis, heartburn, and hemorrhoids. Anti-acid in the gut, blood, and tissues.
Marshmallow root	Treats digestive and respiratory problems by binding to and eliminating gastrointestinal and respiratory acids.
Turmeric	Anti-inflammatory; treats indigestion and gallbladder disease by binding to and eliminating acids.
Peppermint	Treats colicky pain, irritable bowel syndrome, indigestion, gallstones, candida, and yeast infections, and relieves mucous congestion.

Herb	Benefit
Corn silk	Diuretic, rich source of potassium; treats disorders of the urinary tract, liver, kidneys, and bladder.
Couch grass	Treats sore throats, kidney stones, and difficult urination.
Pau d'arco	Immune stimulant, effective against bacterial, fungal, viral, parasitic, and yeast infections.
Rosemary	Potent anti-acid, antiseptic, and antispasmodic. Used for nervous disorders, upset stomach, headaches, pain, strains, and bruises.
Thyme	Antiseptic; treats respiratory and digestive problems. Also treats headaches, asthma, allergies, and coughs.
Black walnut leaf	Treats fungal and parasitic infections, relieves constipation, and may help eliminate warts. Also helps balance blood sugar levels, burns toxins and fatty deposits, and has anticancer effects.
Wintergreen	Treats headaches, arthritis, and muscle pain; reduces inflammation and stimulates circulation.
Celery seed	Reduces blood pressure; treats arthritis, gout, and kidney problems; diuretic and anti-acid properties.
Dandelion	Diuretic, cleans blood and liver from excess acidity, increases bile production, improves kidney, spleen, pancreas, and stomach function.
Lemongrass	Aids in digestion; treats fevers, flu, headaches, and intestinal irritation.
Meadowsweet	Tightens tissues, promotes elimination of excessive fluids, reduces inflammation. Treats colds, flu, nausea, digestive disorders, muscle cramps and aches, and diarrhea.
Papaya	Aids in digestion. Treats heartburn, indigestion, and inflammatory bowel diseases.
Plantain	Diuretic; treats indigestion and heartburn.
Sage	Stimulates central nervous system and digestive tract.
Rose hips	Antioxidant properties; fights inflammation, bacteria, and fungi; relaxes stomach; stimulates circulation and digestion; detoxifies the liver from endogenous acid production.
Parsley	Anti-acid, anticancer effects, stimulates digestion, helps bladder, kidney, liver, stomach, lung, and thyroid function.

Chapter 9

Exercise Right

The Doctor of the Future will give no medicine,
but will involve the patient in the proper use of food,
fresh air, and exercise.
—THOMAS EDISON

There's one last key to ridding yourself of overacidity, sugar intolerances, diabetes, and all their negative consequences. Besides green foods and good fats, green drinks, and nutritional supplements, you need a fitness program to help you get and stay alkaline. Everyone needs exercise, of course, and people with diabetes have an even greater need for it than the general population because they are more sensitive to the increase of acids from sugar metabolism, which exercise helps clear away.

Exercise is important not only for its famous cardiovascular benefits, contributions to strength and flexibility, and ability to improve mood and decrease stress. It isn't just the way it improves blood pressure, triglycerides, and insulin levels that make exercise so crucial for anyone with diabetes or a prediabetic condition.

Exercise is also critical to eliminating acids from the body. Exercise makes you breathe. It makes you sweat. It pumps your lymph system. And this trio, as you'll see in this chapter, is incomparable in cleansing your body. This happens through the lungs and through the skin: respiration and perspiration. Thank goodness for our skin's thirty-five hundred pores per inch! Exercise moves acids through them (in sweat) and through the lungs to keep you in pH balance.

But the way most of us do it, exercise is actually hazardous to health. So is overexercising. So is *not* exercising. Thus, you have to exercise. But you have to do it right.

By explaining key differences between aerobic and anaerobic exercise, how the acid–alkaline balance shifts when you exercise, whether your body burns sugar or fat during exercise, and the role of the lymphatic system—as well as reviewing details on specific types of exercise—this chapter will help you choose the right type of exercise for true and lasting health. You'll get results even from regular brisk walks or ten-minute sessions bouncing on a mini-trampoline, but as you're about to see, you have many more options to choose from in fashioning a plan that's right for you.

ANAEROBIC EXERCISE

The energy required for the body to make any movement at all is created by tiny generators within every cell known as mitochondria. Just as with fuel combustion in a car, the process isn't without its drawbacks—it creates acidic by-products. Just what kind of toxins those by-products are is determined by both the fuel being used and the environment within which that fuel is being burned. Ideally, carbon dioxide—a less toxic acid—is released; often it is the more toxic lactic acid that results. As long as the body is taking in plenty of oxygen, energy is extracted via respiration, yielding, as we all learned sometime in Earth Science class, carbon dioxide, which is excreted through the lungs. Without sufficient oxygen, the process shifts to fermentation, expelling lactic acid into the tissues.

It takes twenty parts oxygen to neutralize one part carbon dioxide and maintain that delicate pH balance of 7.365 in the body. That's why after a race, the runners are usually bent over holding their knees or lying down, gasping for breath: They desperately need the oxygen to neutralize the excess buildup of acid from the race before they pass out, or even die. That's why *you'd* pass out or die if you didn't take a breath for a few minutes, even if you haven't been running for the finish line. We all need plenty of oxygen all the time to keep our bodies healthfully alkaline.

Anaerobic (literally "without oxygen") exercise or overexercise—which is anytime you exercise to the point where you are gasping for that oxygen—leads to increased acidity and blood sugar, stressing the pancreas and putting you on that vicious cycle heading toward diabetes. First your blood sugar actually drops as the sugar is consumed for energy. Then the adrenals kick in to release the hormone adrenaline, which signals the liver and muscles to release their stored sugar (glucogen). This release of sugar provides fuel for energy in the short term, but in a state of oxygen deprivation (during anaerobic or overexercise), the increase of sugar creates even more acid and you have entered the vicious cycle of alternating low and high blood sugars leading toward insulin resistance and Type 2 diabetes. Herein is the explanation for that seeming contradiction, the exerciser who can't lose weight, or even gains it: Without enough oxygen, the body is being forced into self-preservation mode, making cholesterol and holding fat to bind acids, leading to obesity.

Weight lifting is the basic example of anaerobic exercise. Classic calisthenics such as push-ups, chin-ups, and sit-ups fall into the same category. I'd make the list much longer, however, to include many things we think of as aerobic ("with oxygen") that tend to be overdone to the point of being effectively anaerobic, like running, uphill cycling, or using a stair climber.

BURNING SUGAR VERSUS FAT

The problem with anaerobic exercise, or overexercise, is that in the absence of oxygen your cellular metabolism shifts from respiration to fermentation. That means your cells are primarily burning sugar for energy, resulting in an increase of lactic acid. Lactic acid is very toxic. It is what causes the aches and pains you feel during and after exercise—the muscle aches you get after a workout, for example. It is always found in greater concentrations in the body wherever there is irritation, inflammation, or pain (as well as in and around cancerous tumors!).

Burning fat rather than sugar, however, results in half the acid production—and twice the energy. As important as that is in your everyday life, it is even more crucial when it comes to exercise. Exercising properly will allow your body to run on fat metabolism, while moving acids out of your body at the same time. Not only will you minimize acidity, but also you'll increase strength and endurance, improve performance of all bodily functions, and extend both the quality and the quantity of your life.

When you are burning sugar, you'll feel light-headed or dizzy. Your thinking may become cloudy, and you may become agitated or anxiety-ridden. Your hands or feet may tingle or be cold, or you may have burning sensations there or elsewhere in your body. You'll be able to hear yourself breathing—you inhale and exhale through your mouth rather than your nose—and you'll be unable to carry on a conversation while exercising. Your muscles will be tight, your fists balled up, and your brow furrowed, and you may have a knot in your throat. Your sweat may smell like ammonia. Your peripheral vision may narrow, and you may feel disconnected with your environment, even to the point that you don't hear your feet hitting the ground when you're running, for example. You may experience systemic or localized pain. In short, you're not going to feel good!

How you feel when you are burning fat stands in stark contrast. You'll feel peaceful, grounded, connected to your environment, even euphoric. You'll think clearly. You'll breathe quietly and easily, through your nose, and be able to chat while exercising. Your facial expressions will be relaxed and happy, and you will feel more flexible. All your senses will be enhanced. You feel no pain: you're in the zone. And you can put yourself in that "runner's high" state without marathon-style expenditure of energy, with the right diet—and the right type of exercise.

NO PAIN, NO GAIN?

No way! "No pain, no gain" is one of the biggest myths of the fitness industry. When you exercise to exhaustion (and are therefore doing anaerobic exercise), you are creating excess acids, acids that break down cells and cause a rise in blood sugar. For example, the pain you feel with exercise—aches, irritation, inflammation—often comes from the release of lactic acid into the tissues, as the body struggles to maintain its 7.365 pH balance. Exercising to the point of pain is a sure way to stress your body right into disease, including diabetes. If you're experiencing pain, you're overacid and your blood sugar is unstable. (If at any point you do feel any pain or discomfort while exercising, stop immediately, and hydrate yourself with green drink.)

Isabelle's Story

I joined one of the world's premier ballet companies when I was eighteen. I'd take a class in the morning, then rehearse for up to six hours, then put on my stage makeup, stretch and warm up my muscles again, and give it my all in the evening performance. This schedule went on for months at a time.

My third year with the company, at the age of twenty-one, I was diagnosed with juvenile diabetes. I had just begun to be featured in leading roles, my dream come true. But just as I should have been basking in the glow of a blossoming career I'd worked for my whole life, the flowering of my life's passion and love, I was instead dealing with a body that felt a hundred years old.

I had to learn to juggle the demands of being an artist and star athlete while walking the tightrope of taking insulin. I feared losing what I loved most, so I was determined to learn everything I could about health and healing so that I could keep dancing. I had always considered myself health-conscious, a granola-raised kid from California, but the more I read, the more confused I became. One expert said high-carbohydrate diet, another said high-protein. This one flogged one miracle supplement, that one another. I think I tried them all at different times—I could tell you many, many stories. Just learning how to take insulin without overshooting it while I was on stage performing took years to figure out.

The diet I eventually figured out worked best for me was one that emphasized a lot of fresh vegetables, good fats like flax, borage, and olive oil, fresh fish, seeds, and nuts, and organic protein like chicken and eggs. Following this routine kept my blood sugars stable without too many fluctuations during the day. In the event of low blood sugar, I used dried fruit instead of straight sugar.

Balancing my blood sugars and finding the best way to eat was not my only problem. Muscle pains and insomnia plagued me, too. Athletes commonly have to deal with muscle pains, but compounded by the diabetes, I was in constant muscle distress. I found it hard to wind down at night from all the excitement and exertion of the day, and often couldn't sleep. It got worse when I was nervous about certain performances that were especially important.

Six years after my diagnosis, I was promoted to soloist with the company. I danced for another seven years before moving on to teaching ballet and staging the ballets I used to dance. And I still performed on occasion. Because I was not dancing so many hours a day, I no longer had the extreme muscle pain I once did. But the injuries from sixteen years of performing remained, and made themselves known especially at the end of a day of teaching and being on my feet. The insomnia, too, was still part of my life whenever I got too busy or stressed out, or had to travel.

As far as my diet went, I found I now required less protein, and felt good with (what I now know are) alkalizing foods. But even though I loved what I ate (and I ate a lot), and even though I kept my blood sugar in good control, I continually struggled with feelings of not being satisfied.

When I first heard about the pH Miracle plan for controlling diabetes, I thought I was basically doing it already. I didn't think adding a green drink with pH drops to my day was something I needed. But I was open to just about anything that might help (especially coming from someone so aligned with what I had already discovered worked for me), so I decided to give it a try. I started with 1 liter of green drink a day, with drops and soy sprouts powder. The rest, as they say, is history.

The first thing I noticed was the effect on my muscles and soft tissues. Years of pain from injuries and tightness left. After about a week, I noticed that my sleep came easier, and was deeper and more restful, even after a stressful day. The other thing I noticed was that I was satisfied with what I ate in a very deep way. I added in some additional supplements, notably EFAs, and increased my green drink to 2 liters a day, eventually working up to 4 and sometimes 5 liters a day.

My blood sugars continued to improve, and now, for the first time in my life, I understand what real health feels like. I feel like I have searched for this since the day I was diagnosed. I am excited and profoundly grateful every day for the continual changes in my health.

WHY YOU SHOULD CARE ABOUT YOUR LYMPHATIC SYSTEM

You know exercise benefits your heart and lungs and muscles, and of course that is all to the good. But what you probably don't know is that perhaps the biggest benefit of all is to your lymphatic system. The lymphatic system links organs (including the spleen), tissues, and ducts via capillaries to move fluid away from tissues and back into the blood, as well as to boost immunity by moving white blood cells around the body. This is how the body gets rid of debris from cell breakdown. This is how the body gets rid of excess acid.

The lymphatic vessels go pretty much wherever blood vessels go. They are lined with a thin, smooth wall of muscle. You have hundreds of lymph nodes spread out along those vessels, concentrated in the neck, armpit, and groin. Lymph, the clear fluid that bathes the cells of the body, helps deliver nutrients, eliminate wastes, and exchange oxygen and carbon dioxide.

The lymphatic vessels seem to be one-way: Lymph moves forward into the lymph nodes to be filtered. Because the lymphatic system doesn't have the benefit of a big pump the way the circulation system has the heart to move blood around, it depends on pressure changes caused by breathing (especially deep breathing) and muscular activity to stimulate the flow of lymph. So regular exercise is key to keeping this crucial system running smoothly, and moving acids (like lactic acid from overexercise) and yeast, bacteria, and viruses out of the tissues.

A lot of things can block your lymphatic system, prime among them a lack of regular aerobic exercise, and anaerobic exercise and overexercise. Acid foods, sugar, and toxic chemicals such as medications, food additives, and preservatives can cause problems, too. Waste from chemical reactions in the cells and from breakdown of tissues, debris from sugar and protein metabolism, and any by-products that can't be cleared by the bloodstream can also block your lymphatic system. Emotional and psychological issues can have an effect, too. The lymphatic system will slow down due to anger, stress, fatigue, or emotional shock.

When the lymph slows down, the cell ends up suspended in an acidic bath. Fresh oxygen and fuel (whether sugar or fats) can't get to the cell. The unused sugar ferments, creating toxic acids; in the presence of acid and absence of oxygen, microforms start to transform. (Which should be familiar by now as the beginning stages of insulin resistance leading to diabetes.) Furthermore, your body won't work as efficiently, and you'll feel all out of energy. You'll have poor circulation. You'll experience systemic and/or localized pain due to acid buildup. You'll retain fluids—one of your body's strategies for neutralizing acid. And you'll be wide open to degenerative disease such as diabetes.

So get your regular—healthy—exercise! You'll "pump" the lymphatic system, making sure the cells get the fuel they need, keeping them bathed in alkaline fluid, and pulling away any toxins and debris, ensuring a healthier and more energized body.

THE RIGHT EXERCISE

You'll run into a lot of health problems with no exercise, or the wrong kind of exercise. Fortunately, the solution is simple: Exercise right. That generally means low-impact aerobic exercise such as walking, cross-training machines, and rebounding (mini-trampolines); more static exercise like yoga, Pilates, and certain types of weight training; and even "passive exercise" such as sauna and massage. This section will give you an overview of several types of exercise that alkalinize the body. Whatever you do, get at least twenty to thirty minutes a day of activity. You should always consult with your doctor before beginning a new exercise program, particularly if you've been a bit of a couch potato.

Walking

Walking gets the muscles moving enough to increase circulation, pump the lymph, and move acids out of your tissues and out of your body. Like all aerobic exercise, it causes the body to burn fat rather than sugar, and reduces stress on the pancreas.

Walk long enough or far enough to break a sweat—about twenty minutes for a man, and thirty minutes for a woman. (Sweat, being an excellent way to move acids out of the body through the skin, is one of the best reasons to exercise.) Stay relaxed and aware of everything around you as you walk, and breathe in and out through your nose.

Jogging

Jogging offers similar benefits, though it must be done with care so it stays aerobic and does not verge into anaerobic exercise. Jogging should always be pleasurable, and never painful. If you begin to experience any pain while jogging, slow down and walk for a while until the pain subsides. Always breathe in and out through your nose, not your mouth. And be sure to sweat!

Swimming

If you have access to a lap pool, swimming is one of the best forms of aerobic exercise because it is essentially no-impact (one step better than low impact), but moves the muscles—which in turn moves the lymph and reduces acidity.

Cross-Trainers

Also known as elliptical trainers, these machines are very beneficial. They work both your upper and lower body at once, with a movement similar to jogging or walking while holding on to handles moving forward and back. You can adjust not only how long you exercise, but also your speed, distance, resistance (on both arms and legs), intensity, and heart rate, not to mention what kind of "terrain" you cover. I think the Life Fitness Cross-Trainer is the best all-around machine; most good gyms have one. Start out on the lowest settings, and do at least thirty minutes a day.

GREENS AT WEST POINT

In 2001, I conducted a six-month study with the members of the West Point gymnastic team—a collection of fit specimens if ever there was one. Still, all the participants who used green drink experienced an increase in energy and performance, and a decrease in soreness after workouts and meets (meaning less lactic acid buildup) and in recovery time.

Yoga

Yoga contains an element of philosophy and/or spirituality in its program. It's a discipline for the mind and emotions as well as the body, and, in fact, aims to integrate the three into a unified whole. (Some classes focus pretty much exclusively on the physical, though, so you should check out a class before you join to make sure the specific approach appeals to you.) On just the physical plane, yoga is an excellent form of exercise because it emphasizes balance, strength, flexibility, and stamina all at once. It fights fat, too. Furthermore, the breathing exercises involved improve circulation and oxygenation. Research shows that yoga practice is an excellent stress reliever, besides reducing physical tension in the body. It can boost self-esteem, improve concentration, and increase your sense of overall well-being through calming the nervous system. Studies looking specifically at diabetes have found that yoga can help manage the disease.

Pilates

Pilates also aims to integrate mind and body. It works the muscles, including the often overlooked deeper muscles, and focuses on "core strength" (around the abdomen and back). Pilates techniques, which emphasize efficient and graceful movement, are designed to improve alignment and breathing, and increase body awareness, all while simultaneously stretching and strengthening the muscles. For people with diabetes, the stretching and breathing can improve circulation, helping remove acids from sugar metabolism.

Weight Training

This can be an excellent form of exercise, but it must be done correctly or it will do more harm than good. You must work with high intensity but low force, building muscle by doing a small number of very slow and controlled repetitions, using modest amounts of weight or resistance—six to ten reps per exercise. Lift the weight and hold it for fifteen seconds where the most effort is required. When a rep takes considerable effort and you can't manage another, stop! You're done with that exercise and it is time to move on to another. Once you've reached ten reps on any given exercise, increase the intensity by holding the weight for progressively longer times, until you are holding each rep for thirty seconds. Then increase the weight enough so that you're back to fifteen seconds, and build up again from there to ten reps and thirty seconds. This approach is known as static contraction, and entire books have been written on the subject if you want more details. The good news is that you should need the gym for only twenty to thirty minutes at a time for the first couple of weeks of a program like this, and only ten to fifteen minutes a session after that, three times a week.

Your goal shouldn't be how much you can tolerate, but how *little* is required to increase muscle size and strength. The ideal is to forever abandon the macho "no pain, no gain" mantra. Real strength comes from weight lifting *without* pain.

Cellercise

Cellercise is one of the best forms of low-impact aerobics. You might already know it as rebounding—bouncing on a small trampoline—but I like the term *cellercise* (coined by author and inventor David Hall) because this kind of movement is the only one that applies weight and movement to every cell in the body at the same time (rather than isolating specific muscles or muscle groups). Using your own body weight to create resistance, cellercise strengthens muscles, connective tissues, ligaments, and bones, and even tightens and lifts internal organs and skin cells. The up-and-down movement also increases circulation of both blood and lymph, but eliminates 80 percent of the stress on your bones and joints of other major forms of aerobic exercise (while preserving the beneficial weight-bearing aspect that is absent in swimming). It's even good for your digestive system, stimulating the smooth muscles of the intestinal tract, which are otherwise difficult or impossible to exercise.

Cellercise burns calories eleven times faster than walking, five times faster than swimming, and three times faster than running, since all the cells are using energy at the same time. All you need is fifteen minutes twice a day.

BENEFITS OF CELLERCISE

Cellercise is especially useful for people with diabetes, because it helps balance blood sugar and regenerate normal function of the pancreas through detoxing every cell in the body of excess acidity. But that's just the start of a long list of good things cellercise does for your body. Cellercise also:

- Increases balance and coordination.
- Reduces risk of cardiovascular problems (strengthens the heart, lowers resting heart rate, reduces cholesterol and triglyceride levels, increases heart capacity).
- Increases production of red blood cells.
- Boosts white blood cell activity.
- Stimulates lymphatic flow.

- Builds muscles, increasing their vigor and tone as well as their size and strength.
- Stimulates metabolism.
- Increases circulation.
- Brings more oxygen to the tissues.
- Increases thyroid output.
- Expands the body's capacity for fuel storage.
- Improves mental performance.
- Reduces aches and pains (from lack of exercise).
- Reduces headaches and back pains.
- Improves digestion and elimination.
- Improves sleep and relaxation.
- Fights fatigue.
- Eases menstrual discomfort.
- Eliminates excess weight.

PASSIVE EXERCISE

Several passive forms of exercise are also excellent for moving the lymphatic fluids, reducing acidity in the body. These are good options for people who, for whatever reason, can't exercise sufficiently. For the rest of us, they are a good supplement to our regular exercise. You might not get *all* the benefits of aerobic exercise or weight training, but then, most passive exercise is more luxurious. How does a massage or sauna sound, for example? Here are the best passive exercises to help you lower your acidity and stabilize your sugar levels.

Deep Breathing

Deep breathing helps release acidic toxins from the body by increasing lymphatic flow. The first organ that lymph and its toxins reach upon being deposited into the bloodstream is the lungs; deep breathing helps expel the toxins, taking some of the stress off your lymphatic system.

NO SMOKING

It's no news that cigarettes are bad for you, but what you probably don't know is that a big part of the reason why is that smoking releases both sugar and yeast into the blood via the lungs. Of course it also wreaks havoc with your ability to breathe properly, which compromises your ability to move lymph through your body to clear acids.

Acupuncture and Acupressure

These create a positive energy field at the points needled or pressed, increasing blood flow and facilitating healing and regeneration of stressed areas of the body (which could include the pancreas).

Saunas

The radiant heat of an infrared sauna causes a profound sweat, flushing toxic acids and heavy metals from the body. Infrared saunas heat the objects in them—in this case your body—rather than just the air, the way ordinary saunas do. The steam or wet heat of regular saunas can carry negative microforms such as yeast and molds that you breathe in. Dry heat in an infrared sauna is much more comfortable, as well, the way Phoenix at 100 degrees is bearable and Miami at 100 degrees is a misery. There are a host of other benefits; a dry heat infrared sauna also:

- Speeds up metabolic processes, including those in the pancreas.
- Inhibits the development of negative microforms.
- Creates a "fever reaction"—rising body temperature—which removes acidic wastes.
- Increases the number of white blood cells.
- Exercises the heart.
- Reduces blood pressure.
- Dilates blood vessels.
- Relieves pain.
- Speeds healing of sprains, bursitis, arthritis, and circulation problems in the hands and feet.
- Increases blood circulation, and thus the removal of acidic toxins through the pores of the skin.
- Promotes relaxation and creates a sense of well-being.

So look for an infrared sauna; some gyms and spas are installing them. I recommend thirty minutes in the sauna at 140 degrees Fahrenheit. Remember that sweating depletes the body of beneficial minerals, too, so replenish your body with green drink afterward.

Lymphatic Massage

Also known as lymphatic manipulation, this is different from other types of massage in that it is aimed at moving lymph through the body, speeding up the elimination of waste products. The massage therapist pumps the lymph nodes, primarily at the armpit, back of the knee, bend of the arm, and bend of the hip, working in the connective tissue that houses them (tissue that also holds muscles to the bone). Applying pressure to the lymph nodes pushes the lymph therein toward the heart; when pressure is released, the node expands, pulling lymph into it, increasing lymph flow throughout the body—much like the action of priming a lawn mower.

This kind of gentle massage improves circulation and relaxes muscles while it also helps strengthen the immune system, balance hormones, and improve digestion, increasing absorption and use of nutrients. And, of course, it is a terrific stress reducer. Not to mention that being cared for and cosseted provides a feeling of well-being. A lot of these same benefits accrue no matter what kind of massage you get, but no other type will do as much to circulate the lymph.

Shelley has studied lymphatic massage with a person trained by the originator of the method, and practiced it for more than twelve years. She's had excellent results, though they are even better when combined with nutritional therapy. I only wish we were as attuned to the power of lymphatic massage in this country as they are in Europe, where most insurance plans cover it fully, and doctors routinely write prescriptions for it.

LYMPHATIC SUPPORT

Exercise, lymphatic massage, and other activities stir up acids, and green drinks are especially important to help alkalize them, keeping the lymphatic system clean and nutrients and oxygen flowing to the cells.

Anytime your lymphatic system needs extra support, you might want to take additional vitamin A. I recommend using three different sources to ensure complete absorption and improve tolerance: dry, water-dispersible (relatively oil-free) fish liver oil; carotene (from plants); and a variety of plants and herbs containing vitamin A, including wheatgrass, barley grass, oat grass, dandelion, and parsley (green drink). Other nutrients that are helpful in supporting the lymphatic system and eliminating acids are: octacosanol (found in unheated, unrefined wheat germ oil), N,N-dimethylglycine, and superoxide dismutase (SOD).

Take a supplement providing between 25,000 and 50,000 IU of vitamin A and at least 10,000 IU of beta-carotene and fish liver oil. Take one capsule with a green drink or water with pH drops six times a day.

A word of warning: If your body is very acidic, you may feel slug-gish, foggy, fatigued, or nauseated after a lymphatic massage. This is normal—the acids that were stuck in your body are being processed. Have a green drink to facilitate the process, and you'll feel good within twenty-four hours.

Self-massage or **body brushing** (using a brush on dry skin) can provide many of the same benefits as lymphatic massage. Always rub toward the heart. Work the area immediately around the lymph node first, applying pressure toward the node, and work your way out.

Chapter 10

pH Miracle Recipes

"It is clear to me how this way of eating can totally change your life. It's a revelation. A way of looking at the world in a new light. It affects the way we look at ourselves, and disease . . . and how the food we put into our bodies affects everything we do."
—JANE CLAYSON, CBS NEWS

All that you've read to this point wouldn't get you very far without this chapter, which provides the secret to putting this plan into action: delicious recipes for alkaline food. Understanding why it is important to stop eating acidifying foods, and wanting to do so, is all well and good, but then the question remains: What *are* you going to eat? Look no further for the answer. And get your taste buds ready for a treat. They may be dulled currently to the exquisite wonder of nature's bounty, but soon after you switch over to this way of eating they'll be alive to every natural, wholesome flavor it has to offer.

Shelley Redford Young—my wife—put together the recipes in this chapter, and I think you'll be as glad as I am that she is such an original talent in the kitchen. (And, she'd want me to tell you, she never much cared for cooking before we went alkaline, so rest assured there are plenty of quick and easy recipes here, and plenty your family will love.) Shelley developed many of the dishes here, but also included are some of the results of a recipe contest we held.

Who knew there were quite so many alkaline chefs out there, building their own better meals? She and I both want to thank and honor all those who have shared their creations in this way.

Our first book, *The pH Miracle,* contains an extensive recipe section as well (see the box), so if you ever exhaust what's here you have an option for more ideas about eating in harmony with the pH Miracle plan. And we hope *you* will improvise and innovate as you grow more comfortable with preparing food the pH Miracle way.

In this chapter, you'll find sections for Drinks and Shakes; Soups; Salads; Dressings, Dips, and Sauces; Entrées/Side Dishes; and Snacks/Desserts. I've included a number of "transitional" recipes—foods that are not totally alkaline, with ingredients such as tofu or tortillas, meant to get you away from highly acidic foods; you must eat these in moderation. Most of them are winners in the Transitional Recipes Category of our recipe contest, so you'll see right up top that they are. Use the recipe index if you want to find a specific recipe.

RECIPE INDEX

PH MIRACLE RECIPES

The following recipes in this book also appear in *The pH Miracle*:

Popeye Soup
AsparaZincado Soup
Creamy or Crunchy Broccoli Soup
Green Raw Soup
All-Vegetable Cocktail
Healing Soup
Celery Soup
Broccoli/Cauliflower Soup
Creamy Vegetable Soup
Celery Cauliflower Soup
Alfalfa Sprout Salad
Spinach Salad
Colorful Cabbage
Alkalizing Energizing Cucumber Salad
Essential Dressing
Soy Cucumber Dressing
Lime Ginger Sauce

While just about all the recipes in *The pH Miracle* will work on this program, the following recipes will be particularly beneficial to diabetics if you want to look them up:

Gazpacho
Vegetable Minestrone Soup
Chunky Veggie Soup
Zucchini Toss
Spring's Pesto
Broccoli Salad
Bean Sprout Salad
Potassium Salad
Wheat Sprout Salad

Rainbow Salad
Sprouted Lentil Salad
Leprechaun Surprise Dip
Tofu Salad Spread
Herbed Salad Dressing
Herb Oil
Parsley Dressing

RECIPES FOR USE DURING
A LIQUID FEAST OR CLEANSE

RECIPES GOOD FOR RAISING LOW BLOOD SUGAR

DRINKS AND SHAKES

Many of these drinks and shakes can serve as a complete meal. They enter the bloodstream quickly and give the greatest amount of concentrated nutrition and energy with the least amount of digestive stress of anything you could eat.

The Raw Perfection Morning Monster Juice

SERVES 1–2

Donated by Mike Nash.

This is great when you need something that's going to stick with you until midday; the fat will help you feel full. Besides providing that fat, the avocado is the key to the creaminess of this smoothie.

1 package (bunch) kale
1 head celery
1 lemon
Handful of spinach leaves
1 avocado
1 tsp. green powder
1 chili pepper

Put the kale, celery, and lemon through a juicer, then combine in a blender with the remaining ingredients.

AvoRado Kid Super Green Shake

SERVES 1

This is by far our favorite cool green shake, and we've enjoyed it for break-fast, lunch, and dinner, or anytime we want a snack. It's a great way to get the concentrated nutrition and chlorophyll of green powder and soy sprouts powder (and an especially great way to get it into your kids). The cucumber and lime cool the body, and the essential fats in God's great but-ter, avocado, and the soy sprouts make this shake one that you can burn on for many hours.

1 avocado
½ English cucumber
1 tomatillo
1 lime (peeled)
2 cups fresh spinach
2 scoops soy sprouts powder
1 scoop green powder
1 pkg. stevia
6–8 ice cubes

Blend all the ingredients in a blender on high speed to a thick, smooth consistency. Serve immediately.

Variations:
- Add 1 tsp. almond butter for a nuttier flavor.
- Add coconut milk or Fresh Silky Almond Milk (see page 183) for a creamier shake.
- Make a parfait by layering the shake with layers of dehydrated unsweetened coconut; sprinkle some of the coconut on top.
- Substitute a grapefruit or lemon for the lime for a different taste.
- Add 1 Tbs. fresh-grated ginger.
- Add some seasonings that are bottled in oil (without alcohol) for a new exciting twist of flavor.

• In the summer, freeze AvoRado Kid into pops for a cool frozen treat. You can also completely freeze and then partially thaw small portions of the shake, then chop it up to enjoy as a slush.

Very Veggie Shake

SERVES 1–2

Donated by Parvin Moshiri.

1 cup distilled water
¼ cup flaxseed oil or olive oil
2 small cucumbers, sliced
1 cup spinach
2 avocados
⅓ head romaine lettuce
½ cup broccoli
¼ cup cilantro
¼ cup parsley
2 stalks celery, cut into pieces
⅛ cup fresh mint leaves (or 1 tsp. dry)
2 medium limes or 1 lemon
⅛ cup fresh dill (optional)

Place the water in a blender, then add the oil. Turn the blender to low speed and add the remaining ingredients one at a time. When everything is chopped up, turn up the blender to high speed until you get a beautiful, smooth, and creamy green shake.

Zesty Lemon Ginger Shake

SERVES 1

Donated by Karen Rose.

1 lemon, peeled and chopped
2 Tbs. chopped fresh ginger
1 avocado
1 small cucumber
1–2 tsps. soft tofu

Mix all ingredients together in a blender until creamy. Add water if necessary for your desired consistency.

Variation: To make this higher in protein as well as even more lemony, add:

1 lemon or lime
1–2 tsps. soy sprouts powder
1 tsp. green powder
2 tsps. stevia (with fiber)
¼ cup soft tofu
6–8 ice cubes

Paul's Breakfast in a Blender

SERVES 1

Donated by Paul A. Repicky, Ph.D.

This is a chewy sort of breakfast (or anytime) shake that will keep you going for hours.

½ large, nonsweet grapefruit (or 1 small one), outer layer of rind peeled off (the white inner rind is quite nutritious), core and seeds removed
Handful of sprouts (alfalfa, clover, or other)
Handful of fresh spinach
⅓ cup fresh-ground flaxseeds
1–2 Tbs. Udo's oil
2 cups chopped broccoli
½ cup chopped cucumber
1½ cups water

Mix all the ingredients in a blender on medium speed (or higher if you like it smoother).

Adjust quantities to taste; this usually makes 32 to 34 ounces.

Minty Mock Malt

SERVES 2

Donated by Matthew and Ashley Rose Lisonbee.

½ English cucumber
Juice of 1 lime
Juice of 1 grapefruit

1 avocado
1 cup raw spinach
½ can coconut milk
1 tsp. green powder
2 tsps. soy sprouts powder
8–10 pH drops
2–4 sprigs for fresh mint leaves or ½ tsp. mint flavoring
   (no alcohol) (Frontier brand)
14 ice cubes

Combine all the ingredients in a blender and blend to your desired consistency.

Variation: Leave out the ice cubes, and freeze the malt into pops.

Chi's Green Drink

SERVES 2

Donated by Jill Butler, from her friend
Ernesto Chi Ciccarelli.

1 head romaine or Boston lettuce (use the greenest leafy parts,
   omitting the really light green stems if you wish)
3 cloves garlic
1 lemon
¾ cup water
½ cup olive oil
1 piece cut fresh ginger (optional)
Dash of sea salt
Dash of cayenne pepper
1 cucumber, peeled
½–1 cup steamed broccoli (or use whatever combination of green
   veggies you like—experiment!)

A combination of all or one or none of the following:
2–4 basil leaves, or to taste
¼ cup parsley, or to taste
⅛–¼ cup watercress (leaves only), or to taste

Blend all the ingredients in a blender until smooth.

Carrot Crunch

SERVES 1

Donated by Randy Wakefield.

½ tsp. green powder
7 pH drops
1 cup fresh carrot juice
1 chopped carrot
4 ice cubes

Combine all the ingredients in electric or hand blender and blend until smooth. Serve sprinkled with nutmeg.

✳ All-Vegetable Cocktail

SERVES 2

1 pt. fresh tomatoes
½ tsp. garlic
1 cucumber, sliced
1 green pepper
Sprigs of fresh parsley
¼ onion, sliced

2–3 lettuce leaves
½ tsp. ginger

Blend all the ingredients in a blender on low speed.

Fresh Silky Almond Milk

SERVES 4–6 (MAKES APPROXIMATELY 1 QUART)

4 cups fresh raw almonds
Pure water
Nylon stocking (for straining)

Soak the fresh raw almonds overnight in a bowl of water. Drain. Place the almonds in a blender until it is a third full (about 2 cups), then add the pure water to fill the blender. Blend on high speed until you have a white creamy-looking milk. Take a nylon stocking (I use a *clean* white knee-high nylon stocking) and pour the mixture through it over a bowl or pan, then let it drain. Squeeze with your hand to get the last of the milk through the nylon. (The solids you strain out can be used in the shower as a great body scrub.) Thin with water to your desired consistency. Drink as is, or add a bit of stevia to sweeten it. You can also use it in soups, shakes, or puddings. Almond milk will stay fresh for about 3 days in the refrigerator.

SOUPS

Soups are especially great for diabetics: Because they are liquid, they enter the bloodstream quickly.

Think of soup as a breakfast food now that you are avoiding the conventional starchy, sugar, and high-protein options.

Navy Bean Soup

SERVES 4–6

Donated by Roxy Boelz.
Third place, pH Miracle Recipe Contest.

1 cup adzuki beans, soaked overnight
1 cup navy beans, soaked overnight
1 small onion, chopped
2 large carrots, grated
RealSalt to taste
2 tsps. grated fresh ginger
1 cup chopped celery
Nutmeg or cardamom

Cook the beans till just tender. Cool slightly. If necessary, add water to get the consistency of soup you want. Add the onion, carrots, salt, and ginger. Transfer to a food processor or blender and process to the texture desired. You can add the celery with the ingredients to be blended, or afterward for crunchiness. Serve sprinkled with nutmeg, cardamom, or a spice of your choice.

Tortilla Soup

SERVES 4–6

Donated by Cheri Freeman.
Third place, pH Miracle Recipe Contest,
Transitional Recipes Category.

Some people like to use organic chicken broth instead of veggie. This soup, minus tortillas and tofu, would be great for a liquid feast.

Sprouted-grain tortillas (½ for each serving) (optional)
3 cups yeast-free vegetable broth (read the label; Morga and Pacific brands have no yeast)
1 cup pureed fresh tomatoes, or packaged strained tomatoes with no preservatives or additives
8 oz. baked seasoned tofu, sliced or coarsely chopped
2–3 tsps. olive oil
2 Tbs. chopped garlic
2 jalapeños, seeded and chopped very fine
½ onion, chopped very fine
½ cup cilantro, chopped very fine
RealSalt to taste
Garlic pepper blend to taste
1 avocado, diced

Preheat the oven to 200 degrees. Place your tortillas directly on the baking rack until they are crisp, about 10 to 20 minutes. Pour the broth and tomato puree into a saucepan and begin heating on very low heat while preparing the vegetables and tofu. In a small skillet, brown the tofu in the olive oil. Add to the broth. Add garlic, jalapeños, onion, and spices. When the mixture is warmed, turn off the heat and add the avocado. Serve with broken bits of tortilla sprinkled on top for some added crunch.

Vegan Chili

SERVES 2–4

Donated by Cheri Freeman.
Third place, pH Miracle Recipe Contest,
Transitional Recipes Category.

Great on cold nights!

2 soy veggie burger patties, crumbled (Boca brand is good)
¼ cup olive oil
½ onion, chopped
1 jalapeño, chopped (with or without seeds, depending on how
    hot you want it)
1 Tbs. chili powder
1 tsp. RealSalt
2 cloves garlic, chopped
3 cups strained tomatoes
2 cups tossed salad (mixed greens, chopped red and yellow pep-
    pers, chopped carrots, etc.)
Vegan cheese shreds (optional)

In a saucepan or cast-iron pot, brown the crumbled patties in the olive oil. Add all the remaining ingredients except the salad and cheese (if you're using this). Adjust the seasonings to your own taste. If you don't like it too hot, you can seed your jalapeño. Put about half the chili in a blender, add the salad mix, and puree. Pour this back into the chili and stir thoroughly. Serve topped with vegan cheese.

French Gourmet Puree

SERVES 6

Donated by Eric Prouty.
Second place, pH Miracle Recipe Contest.

This is a beautiful, soothing alkaline puree. Sometimes I like to double the amount of lettuce to thin it out a bit.

1 avocado
2 stalks celery
1 head romaine lettuce
1 small tomato
1 handful spinach
1 small cucumber, peeled
2 cloves garlic
⅓ onion
2 Tbs. olive oil
Herbes de Provence
Sprouts (optional)

Puree all the vegetables with a juicer, doing the onion last. Mix in the olive oil, then Herbes de Provence to taste. Serve with sprouts sprinkled on top.

Creamy Watercress Soup

SERVES 4–6

Donated by Deborah Johnson.

2 cups pure water
1 cauliflower (cut into 1-inch pieces)
2 cups vegetable broth

2 cups chopped fresh watercress (reserve a sprig or two for gar-
    nish)
1 cup zucchini pieces
1 cup broccoli pieces
1 cup celery pieces
4 green onions, tops removed
¼ cup extra-virgin olive oil
RealSalt to taste

Boil the water, remove from the heat, add the cauliflower, and allow
to rest for 5 minutes. Place the cauliflower and water in a food
processor or blender and process until smooth. Add the remaining
ingredients and blend until your desired consistency is reached. Do
not overblend. Serve warm or chilled. Garnish with a sprig of watercress.

Clean and Simple Soup

SERVES 1–2

Donated by Eric Prouty.
Second place, pH Miracle Recipe Contest,
Alkalarian Recipes Category.

1 cucumber, cubed
1 avocado, cubed
Mint (optional)

Place the ingredients in a food processor with an S blade. Mix until
almost smooth. Serve garnished with mint leaf.

Soothing Cooling Tomato Soup

SERVES 2

The combination of fresh tomatoes and avocado makes this silky-smooth cooling soup high in lycopene and lutein.

6 medium tomatoes, juiced and strained (pour through a fine-mesh strainer or nylon knee-high stocking)
½ avocado
¾ cup fresh coconut water (make sure this is fresh, taken from a coconut)
1 cucumber, juiced
RealSalt to taste
Stevia (optional)

Blend all the ingredients until smooth. For a sweeter soup, add stevia to taste.

Cool Raw Red Soup

SERVES 2–4

This is a raw soup made by juicing all your veggies and then blending them with avocado and some clear fresh coconut water. It has a cooling effect, and is light and refreshing—perfect for a hot summer day.

1 beet
½ large English cucumber
4 stalks celery
1–2 carrots
1 small clove garlic
¼ cup fresh cilantro
½ avocado

¼ cup fresh coconut water (which should be clear and slightly sweet)
Grated veggies (for garnish)

Juice the first six ingredients, then pour the juice through a clean knee-high nylon stocking or a fine-wire-mesh strainer. Mix in a blender with the avocado and coconut water. Garnish if desired with grated veggies.

Roasted Leek Ginger Soup

SERVES 4

1 leek, thoroughly cleaned and cut into ⅓-inch slices
1 tsp. fresh ginger, cut into thin slices
1–2 Tbs. olive or grape seed oil
1 cup freshly strained Fresh Silky Almond Milk (see the recipe on page 183)
2 cups vegetable broth
½–1 tsp. RealSalt

In a soup pot, stir-fry the leek and ginger in the oil until softened and browned on the edges. Pulse-chop the leek and ginger in a food processor and return to the soup pot. Add the almond milk, broth, and RealSalt. Warm and serve.

Variation: Add garlic with the leeks and ginger, and stir in diced roasted bell peppers.

Potato Vegetable Soup

SERVES 4

Donated by Terry Douglas.

This is a nice full-bodied veggie soup.

4–6 small red potatoes
1 medium yellow onion, chopped
1–2 Tbs. olive oil
2 cloves garlic, chopped
2 cans vegetable broth
1 stalk celery, sliced
2 carrots, sliced into rounds
Salt, pepper, and cayenne
1–2 cups baby spinach leaves
½ inch fresh ginger, sliced or julienned
Bragg Liquid Aminos (optional)
Basil (optional)
Few leaves of cilantro
½ cucumber, chopped
1 tomato, chopped
½ green or red pepper, chopped

Cook the potatoes in boiling water until tender (about 20 minutes). In a separate soup pot, over low heat, sauté the onion in the olive oil; add the garlic when the onion is almost done. Add the broth, celery, and carrots. If you don't have lots of liquid, add a can of water. Heat until warm, 3 to 5 minutes; the veggies should still be crunchy. Season to taste with salt, pepper, and cayenne. Remove from the heat. Add the spinach and ginger. To serve, quarter the potatoes and divide them among four soup bowls. (Optional: Add a drop of Bragg Liquid Aminos and a basil leaf in each bowl.) Add soup, and top with cilantro, cucumber, tomatoes, and pepper. Serve immediately, with crackers or sliced avocado.

Spicy Latin Lentil Soup

SERVES 4

Donated by Cathy Galvis.

6 cups water
2 cups lentils
2 carrots (sliced)
¼ tsp. cayenne pepper
⅛ tsp. black pepper
1 tsp. Bragg Liquid Aminos
2 bay leaves
1 onion (chopped)
2 cloves garlic (minced)
½ green pepper (chopped)
½ red bell pepper (chopped)
1 stalk celery (chopped)
½ tsp. seeded and chopped jalapeño pepper
1 tsp. olive oil
¼ cup chopped cilantro

In a large pot, add the water and lentils and bring to a boil. Add the carrots, cayenne pepper, black pepper, Bragg, and bay leaves. Return to a simmer and cover. In a separate pan, sauté the onion, garlic, green and red peppers, celery, and jalapeño pepper in the olive oil for a few minutes. Set aside. Cook the lentils for approximately 20 minutes and add the sautéed onions and peppers. Cook for 10 more minutes, or until the lentils are soft. Serve garnished with the cilantro.

✳ Creamy Tomato Soup ✳

SERVES 2

Donated by Gladys Stenen.

4 roma tomatoes (or equivalent)
2 green onion tips (using about 1 inch of white/light
    green part)
¼ green pepper
1 cup vegetable broth
1 avocado or ¼ pkg. soft tofu
1 tsp. sea salt
Pepper to taste

Liquefy all the ingredients in a blender. Heat just to warm.

Creamy Cauliflower Confetti Soup

SERVES 6–8

This soup is deceptively creamy—you'd think it had dairy in it. The roasted veggie bits provide the confetti appearance. Sprinkle roasted bell peppers over the top and a dash of Zip seasonings for more color.

1 head cauliflower
3 yellow crookneck squash
4 zucchinis
2 yellow onions
2 pks. cherry tomatoes
½ celery root
8 cloves garlic
¼–½ cup grape seed oil
1 qt. Fresh Silky Almond Milk (see page 183)
4 cups vegetable broth

Preheat the oven to broil. Cut the veggies into bite-sized pieces, place them on nonstick cookie sheets, and rub with the grape seed oil. Broil until lightly browned, 10 to 15 minutes. While the veggies are roasting, prepare the almond milk and place it in a soup pot. When the veggies are done, add the cauliflower to a blender with half the onion and half the celery root and blend with enough of the almond milk to get a rich and creamy consistency. Place the mixture in a soup pot. Pulse-chop the remaining veggies in a food processor until minced and add them to the soup. Stir to separate the bits. Add the broth and stir well.

Scrap Soup

SERVES 4

Donated by Mary Seibt.

3 large carrots
2 stalks celery
6 cups distilled water
4 tsps. instant vegetable broth (yeast-free)
1 large yellow onion
4 stalks asparagus, chopped
1½ tsps. cumin
2 tsps. dill
RealSalt to taste
2 tsps. 21 Spice Salute or Zip

Shred the carrots and celery in a food processor. Bring the water to a boil, adding the vegetable broth and onion. Once boiling, turn off the heat. Add the carrots, celery, and asparagus and let stand until the vegetables are tender. Cool enough to put in a blender and mix all the ingredients. Serve warm.

Veggie Almond Chowder

SERVES 4

This soup is even better after it has set in the refrigerator overnight and the flavors have blended.

3 cups soaked almonds (blanch to remove skins if desired) or 2–4
    cups Fresh Silky Almond Milk (see page 183)
Juice of 1–2 lemons
1 garlic clove
1 tsp. Garlic Herb Bread Seasoning (Spice Hunter)
1 qt. vegetable broth (I use Pacific brand)
2 tsps. dehydrated tomato powder (Spice House)
1 tsp. RealSalt
½ tsp. cumin
½ tsp. celery salt
Black pepper or Zip to taste (Spice Hunter)
¼ tsp. green Thai curry paste
1 head broccoli
1 yellow onion
2–3 stalks celery
½ pound fresh green peas (from the pod)

Put the first eleven ingredients (up through the curry paste) in a blender and blend until very smooth. Place in a soup pot. Steam or steam-fry the veggies, and add to the soup pot. Warm and serve.

Tera's Any-Meal Veggie Soup

SERVES 6

Donated by Tera Prestwich.

1 medium onion
3 cloves garlic (1 tsp. minced)
5–7 sun-dried tomatoes
2–3 Tbs. Bragg Liquid Aminos
1 Tbs. parsley (¼ cup fresh)
2 tsp. RealSalt
Pepper to taste (I use 1 tsp.)
1 qt. vegetable broth
1 qt. water
1 head cauliflower
1 bunch broccoli
1 bunch celery (I use the leaf also)
1 lb. carrots
½ lb. fresh green beans
½ lb. peas

Blend the first seven ingredients (through the pepper) in a food processor. Put into a soup pot and cook until the onion is clear. Add the broth and water and bring to a boil. Chop the veggies (and feel free to get creative by including any veggies you like, instead of or in addition to the ingredients above), and add to the soup along with more water if necessary. Cook until the veggies are just tender but still a little crunchy.

Celery Root Soup

SERVES 4

Celery root (or celeriac) is the bulb root of the celery stalk. It is a large, gnarly, rough-skinned root. Not the most attractive of vegetables sitting in the produce section, but nonetheless delicious and very good for you. Wash celery root thoroughly with a brush to loosen dirt trapped in the gnarls. It is somewhat difficult to peel, so break out a good sharp knife or trusty peeler.

2 white onions, chopped
1–2 Tbs. grape seed oil
1 large celery root, peeled and chopped into large bite-sized
    chunks
1 cup water or vegetable broth
RealSalt to taste

Sauté the onions in the oil until softened and lightly browned. Add the celery root and water and steam for 5 to 10 minutes, until the veggies are done. Put the soup in a blender with enough water or broth to cover the top of the onions and celery root. Blend until smooth and creamy. Add more water if necessary to reach your desired consistency, and season to taste with RealSalt. Serve warm as a soup, or spoon over veggies as a sauce or gravy. Experiment with adding your favorite seasonings.

Creamy Curry Broccoli Soup

SERVES 2

Donated by Dr. Gladys Stenen.

2 cups broccoli
2 cups vegetable broth (adjust the amount to reach your desired
thickness)
¼ pkg. soft tofu (or more to taste)
1 tsp. curry powder
Salt and pepper to taste

Liquefy all the ingredients in a blender, then warm.

Special Celery Soup

SERVES 6–8

*This is a perfect soup to serve as an appetizer before your main course, or
on a day when you're tired and need to give your mind, body, and digestive tract a rest.*

1 whole head celery, including core and leaves, sliced
1 leek (sliced white part)
1 Tbs. grated ginger
1 Tbs. coconut oil
1 qt. Fresh Silky Almond Milk (see page 183)
Vegetable broth (optional)

Sauté the celery, leek, and ginger in the oil until softened. Place half
in the blender with half the almond milk and blend well. Mix with
the remaining veggies and almond milk, and warm. Thin with vegetable broth if desired.

Green Gazpacho Two Ways

SERVES 4–6

Donated by Eric Prouty.
Second place, pH Miracle Recipe Contest.

You can prepare this soup simply for a refreshing taste, or you can make it robust with the addition of herbs (which is what my family prefers). Either way, it's a wonderfully alkaline soup, packed with chlorophyll.

6 roma tomatoes
1 head romaine lettuce
2 green bell peppers
1½ large (or 2 average-sized) English cucumbers
½ red onion
2 avocados
3 cloves garlic
¼ cup fresh lemon juice
¼ tsp. RealSalt
2 Tbs. olive oil
1½ tsps. basil
½ tsp. dill
¼ tsp. oregano
⅛ tsp. sage powder

Chop all the vegetables. Mix the avocado, garlic, and lemon juice in a food processor (with an S blade) until smooth, and empty into a bowl. Process the tomatoes and romaine until smooth, and add to the bowl. Pulse the peppers, cucumbers, and onion until chunky (approximately ⅛ to ¼ inch) and empty into the bowl. Mix well with salt and olive oil, and add the herbs if desired.

Tofu Vegetable Soup

SERVES 4–6

Donated by Jennifer Grinberg.

1 32-oz. container Pacific-brand organic vegetable broth
2 leeks, cut lengthwise, cleaned, and chopped small
1 large onion, quartered
1 pkg. fresh firm tofu, drained and cut into small cubes
1 large bok choy, sliced small
4–5 stalks celery, chopped
½ lb. fresh snow peas, ends cut
½ tsp. freshly chopped gingerroot (optional)
RealSalt and freshly ground pepper
2–3 scallions, chopped small (for garnish)
Dash of cayenne (optional)

Pour the vegetable broth into a medium cooking pot. Place the leeks and quartered onion into the broth and simmer while preparing the other ingredients. You can add additional water if the taste of the broth is too strong. Place the remaining ingredients into the broth and simmer until the bok choy softens. Serve in individual bowls and garnish with the scallions and cayenne, if desired.

Popeye Soup

SERVES 4–6

This is a wonderful alkalizing soup because of the cucumbers and greens. It is ready in just 10 minutes. Serve warm with a fresh tortilla for dipping.

1 avocado
1 cup water or vegetable broth (Pacific Foods of Oregon brand is
   yeast-free)

2 cucumbers, unwaxed
1 cup fresh raw spinach
2 green onions
1 clove garlic
⅓ red bell pepper
Bragg Liquid Aminos or RealSalt to taste
Middle Eastern spices: ½–1 tsp. Spice Hunter Garam Masala;
 ½–1 tsp. Curry Seasoning; and ½ tsp. Zip
Fresh lime juice, to taste
4 spearmint leaves (for garnish)

In a Vita-Mix or blender, add the avocado and half the water or broth and puree, then add the rest of the veggies one at a time, blending to your desired thickness and thinning with the remaining water if desired. Add the Bragg Aminos or RealSalt to taste, and flavor with spices and lime juice as desired. You might add a couple of minced sun-dried tomatoes, too. Experiment! This soup is good while on a liquid feast.

Warming options: This soup can be served warm or cold. If you're blending it in a Vita-Mix, the longer you blend, the warmer the soup will get. If you do not have a Vita-Mix, you can carefully warm the soup (not cook it) in an electric or stovetop skillet on low heat. Warm the soup only until you can hold your finger in it without having to pull it out—about 118 degrees, which will keep the food warm but still raw. Serve with spearmint leaves on top. Enjoy!

AsparaZincado Soup

SERVES 3–5

This great soup is rich in zinc and has a rich tomato flavor—and takes only 15 minutes to prepare.

12 stalks medium asparagus (or 17 stalks thin)
5–6 large tomatoes
1 cup fresh parsley
3–5 sun-dried tomatoes (bottled in olive oil)
¼ cup dried onion
4 cloves fresh garlic
1 red bell pepper
1–2 tsp. Spice Hunter Herbes de Provence
2 tsp. Spice Hunter Deliciously Dill
1 avocado
Bragg Liquid Aminos to taste
2 lemons or limes, cut into thin slices (for garnish)

Trim and dice the tips from the asparagus and set aside for garnish. In a food processor or Vita-Mix, blend the asparagus and red tomatoes, parsley, dried tomatoes, onion, garlic, red bell pepper, and spices. Then blend in the avocado until the soup is smooth and creamy. Season with Bragg to taste. Warm in an electric skillet and garnish with lemon or lime slices on top, or serve cold in the summertime. Sprinkle the diced asparagus tips on top of the soup just before serving. Yummy!

Green Raw Soup

SERVES 4–6

This is a wonderfully alkalizing soup that I prefer served cold in the summer months and warmed in the winter. It's energizing and easy to digest.

1–2 avocados
1–2 cucumbers, peeled and seeded
1 jalapeño pepper, seeded
Juice of ½ lemon
1–2 cups light vegetable broth or water
3 cloves roasted garlic
1 Tbs. fresh cilantro
1 Tbs. fresh parsley
½ yellow onion, diced
1 carrot, finely diced

Puree all the ingredients (except the onion and carrot) in a food processor or Vita-Mix. Use more or less water for your desired consistency. Add the onion and raw crunchy carrot bits at the end for a garnish. Yum!

Healing Soup

Serves 6–8

This soup is good anytime. It is soothing when you are tired or stressed, or if you have a cold or flu, and is very antifungal.

2–3 whole cloves garlic
1 large whole onion
2–3 qts. water
3 Tbs. yeast-free instant vegetable broth
1 cucumber
1–2 carrots (optional)
1 small head cabbage or broccoli (optional)
2 stalks celery (optional)
2–3 Tbs. diced fresh ginger
2 Tbs. fresh cilantro
RealSalt to taste

Crush the garlic cloves and lightly steam-fry. Set aside. Put the whole onion in water in a deep pan and simmer until it's transparent (approximately 1 hour). Add the garlic and vegetable broth. Slice the cucumber and any of the optional veggies you are using, and add to the soup. Simmer 10 to 15 minutes. Add the ginger, cilantro, and salt, adjusting to taste.

Variation 1: You could also bring the water to a boil, then take it off the burner and drop in assorted finely chopped veggies. This would just warm, but not cook the vegetables.

Variation 2: You can grate, juice, or process the ingredients into a wet paste and then add them to hot water.

Celery Soup

SERVES 2

4–5 stalks celery (including leaves, if fresh)
3 cups pure water
2 Tbs. yeast-free instant vegetable broth
Flaxseed oil, to taste
Bragg Liquid Aminos, to taste
Cayenne pepper, to taste

Steam-fry the celery in a little water until tender. Add the water and broth mix. Pour all into a blender, and blend for 15 to 20 seconds. Reheat, adding the flaxseed oil, Bragg Liquid Aminos, and cayenne pepper to taste, and serve.

Broccoli/Cauliflower Soup

SERVES 4

⅓ cup soaked almonds
1 cup cucumber juice or vegetable broth
1 clove garlic, minced
1–2 cups chopped broccoli
1–2 cups chopped cauliflower
¼ tsp. cumin
¼ tsp. curry powder
1 Tbs. lemon or lime juice
1 Tbs. Bragg Liquid Aminos
½ tsp. RealSalt

In a food processor or blender, combine the almonds with the cucumber juice or broth and the garlic. Blend well. With the machine still running, add the broccoli and cauliflower and blend until smooth. Finally, blend in the seasonings and lemon or lime juice, Bragg Aminos, and salt. Add more broth or water to reach your desired consistency.

Variation: Use an avocado instead of the almonds and use this recipe for a salad dressing.

Creamy Vegetable Soup

SERVES 8

This rich soup gets its creaminess from tofu. Be sure to blend it thoroughly (I think the blender is best) so you get a rich, even, smooth, creamy texture.

1 cup chopped onion
2 cloves garlic, minced
3 stalks celery, chopped

2 cups shredded green cabbage
½ lb. asparagus, cut small
2 large leeks, chopped
4 cups vegetable broth
2 Tbs. chopped fresh parsley
2 tsps. dried dill
2 tsps. dried basil
1 tsp. dried oregano
RealSalt and pepper, to taste
1 pkg. soft tofu

In a skillet, steam-fry the onion and garlic for a few minutes. Add the celery, cabbage, and asparagus. Transfer to a large pot and add the leeks and vegetable broth. Stir in the parsley, dill, basil, oregano, salt, and pepper. Simmer just to brighten the veggies. Let cool a bit, then puree in a blender or food processor 2 cups at a time with some of the tofu, and return to another pot. Heat the soup no higher than 118 degrees, and serve.

Celery/Cauliflower Soup

SERVES 6–8

1 onion, peeled and chopped
1 Tbs. oil (olive or Udo's)
1 whole head celery, trimmed and chopped (save some celery leaves for garnish)
1 head cauliflower, trimmed and chopped
1–2 qts. vegetable broth
½–1 qt. Fresh Silky Almond Milk (see page 183)
Salt, pepper, and seasonings of choice, to taste

Steam-fry the onion in a little water and oil in a large soup pan for about 5 minutes without browning. Pulse-chop the celery and cauliflower in the food processor until finely chopped.

Add the celery and cauliflower mix to the pan and warm until tender. Add the vegetable broth and almond milk and simmer for 15 to 30 minutes—or you can leave this raw and not cook at all.

Puree the soup mixture in a blender or food processor until a smooth texture is achieved. Season with salt and other seasonings of choice. Serve warm or cold.

Creamy or Crunchy Broccoli Soup

SERVES 4–6

This high-protein soup is a must for broccoli lovers! And it takes just 15 minutes to prepare.

2 cups vegetable broth or water
3–4 cups chopped broccoli
1 red bell pepper, chopped
2 red or yellow onions, chopped
1 avocado
1–2 stalks celery, cut in large pieces
Bragg Liquid Aminos or RealSalt to taste
Cumin and ginger, to taste (experiment with different spices!)

In an electric skillet, warm the broth or water, keeping the temperature at or below 118 degrees (finger test). Add the chopped broccoli and warm for 5 minutes. In a blender, puree the warmed broccoli, bell pepper, onions, avocado, and celery, thinning with additional water if necessary to achieve the preferred consistency. If desired, save the broccoli stalks (peeling off the tough outer skin), process them in a food processor until they are small chunks, and toss into the soup just before serving to add crunch!

Serve warm, flavoring with Bragg, fresh ginger, cumin, or any other spices you like. Add a slice of lemon on top to garnish.

SALADS

Salad is the most important part of a meal, especially for someone with diabetes. It is alkaline, high in water, and high in fiber, and should take up the major portion of your plate (70 to 80 percent).

Lentil–Brazil Nut Salad

SERVES 1–2

Donated by Roxy Boelz.
Third place, pH Miracle Recipe Contest.

1½ cups lentils, cooked
1 cup edamame (soybeans), shelled
1 cup spinach, rinsed and chopped
¼ lime juice
Dash of RealSalt
½–1 tsp. fresh ginger
2–3 Tbs. chopped Brazil nuts
Sprinkle of parsley

Combine the lentils, edamame beans, and spinach. Combine the lime juice, salt, and ginger, and stir into the bean mixture. Sprinkle with Brazil nuts and parsley.

Lemony Green Bean Salad

SERVES 1–2

Donated by Roxy Boelz.
Third place, pH Miracle Recipe Contest.

1 cup cut green beans
1 cup sliced zucchini
½ cup sliced daikon (radish)
Juice of 1 lemon
½ cup dulse flakes
½ cup cut parsley

Lightly steam the green beans. Cool. Combine with the zucchini and daikon. Stir in the lemon juice. Sprinkle with the dulse flakes and parsley.

Moroccan Mint Salad

SERVES 4–6

Donated by Lisa El-Kerdi.
Best in Show, pH Miracle Recipe Contest.

The perfect accompaniment to North African Bean Stew, page 256.

1 bunch parsley, stems removed
1 bunch mint, stems removed
½–1 jalapeño
2 cucumbers, seeded and minced by hand
4–6 scallions, minced by hand
4 tomatoes, seeded and finely chopped
½ cup lemon juice
¼ cup olive oil

½ tsp. RealSalt
½ tsp. paprika

Mince the herbs and jalapeño in a food processor or by hand. Mix in a bowl with the cucumbers and scallions. Add the tomatoes. Stir in the lemon juice, olive oil, and spices. *Sahateck* (to your health)!

Moroccan Coleslaw

SERVES 4–6

Donated by Eric Prouty.
Second place, pH Miracle Recipe Contest.

½ green cabbage
½ red cabbage
⅓ cup fresh lemon juice
1½ tsps. Chinese five-spice powder
1 tsp. caraway seeds
4 Tbs. olive oil

Shred the cabbage in food processor with a shredder wheel. Mix all the ingredients well in a bowl. Let sit for at least half an hour before serving to allow the flavors to blend and the seeds to soften.

More Peas Please

SERVES 4

Donated by Dianne Ellsworth.

4 oz. pea pods, washed, trimmed, and cut into bite-sized pieces
4 oz. pea shoots, 4 inches long, cut in half (or pea sprouts 2 inches long)

10 oz. frozen baby peas, thawed
½ small red onion, sliced very thin, with slices cut in half
2 cloves garlic, pressed through a garlic press or minced finely
¾ cup raw pumpkin seeds
2 Tbs. fresh baby dill weed
2 Tbs. freshly grated ginger
Zest of ½ lemon, cut into ½-inch pieces
Juice of 1 lemon
3 Tbs. olive oil
2 Tbs. grape seed oil
1 Tbs. Udo's oil
½ tsp. dried dill weed
½ tsp. Spice Hunger Garlic Herb Bread Seasoning
Bragg Liquid Aminos to taste

Mix the first nine ingredients (through the lemon zest) in a salad bowl. Make a dressing by mixing the remaining ingredients together thoroughly. Pour half of the dressing over the vegetable mixture and toss well. Add more dressing to taste.

Alkalarian Coleslaw

SERVES 4–6

Donated by Sheila Mack.
Third place, pH Miracle Recipe Contest.

½ head green cabbage, shredded
2 medium carrots, shredded
½ small red onion, sliced thinly into strips
½ cup chopped Italian parsley
1 cup coconut milk (make it fresh by blending the water and meat of a coconut in a blender)
1 tsp. arrowroot powder (optional)
½ tsp. sea salt or to taste

¼ tsp. celery seeds
½ Tbs. fresh lime juice
2 Tbs. grape seed oil
Dash of cayenne pepper
Stevia (optional)

Toss the first four ingredients (through the parsley) in a bowl. Blend the coconut milk and arrowroot (if needed to thicken) in a blender. Blend in the remaining ingredients and toss with the cabbage mixture. This tastes best if you let it sit and chill for a while before serving, to give the flavors a chance to blend.

Popeye Salmon Salad

SERVES 4

Donated by Maraline Krey.
Second place, pH Miracle Recipe Contest.

This salad would also be delicious without the fish! To get the most juice out of the lemon and limes, roll them on the counter before cutting and squeezing them.

1½ lbs. salmon fillet
Juice of 1 lemon
Juice of 3 limes, divided
4 oz. water
2 oz. avocado oil or extra-virgin olive oil
RealSalt
Ground pepper
1 oz. ground flaxseeds
1 oz. poppy seeds
Handful of pine nuts (optional)
1 lb. spinach leaves
½ cup basil leaves

1 cup diced hearts of palm
1 cup diced carrots (optional)
1 cup diced celery (optional)
1 cup diced tomato (optional)
1 cup diced asparagus (optional)

Place the salmon in a glass baking dish. Marinate in the water and the juice of 1 lemon and 1 lime for 2 hours, turning over after an hour.

Preheat the oven to 400 degrees. Bake the salmon in the liquid for 25 minutes, then place under the broiler for 5 minutes to brown the top.

Make the dressing by combining the remaining lime juice, oil, salt and pepper, seeds, and pine nuts, if desired. Use kitchen scissors to cut the spinach and basil leaves into bite-sized pieces. Add into a large salad bowl with whichever of the diced vegetables you choose. Toss with the dressing and let sit until the salmon is ready. To serve, cover dinner plates with salad, and top with pieces of salmon.

Rustic Guacamole (page 238) makes an excellent accompaniment.

Quinoa Salad

SERVES 4

Donated by Charlene Gamble.

Quinoa is a versatile grain. Small and lacy, it makes a good substitute for rice.

½ cup brown rice
1 cup water
½ cup quinoa
1 cup vegetable broth
1 tsp. cumin, divided
1 can (15 oz.) black beans, drained, rinsed, and drained again
1½ red peppers, finely diced

⅓ cup minced cilantro
1½ bunches green onion, chopped
2 stalks celery, chopped
4 Tbs. fresh lime juice
3 Tbs. olive oil (or whatever healthy oil you prefer)
Vege-Sal or RealSalt to taste

In a small saucepan, combine the rice, water, and ½ tsp. cumin. Bring to a boil, cover, reduce the heat, and simmer for 35 minutes. Rinse the quinoa in a sieve. In another small saucepan, combine with the broth and ½ tsp. cumin. Bring to a boil, cover, reduce the heat, and simmer for 15 to 20 minutes. Combine the cooled grains in a bowl with the remaining ingredients. Refrigerate for a while before serving to blend the flavors.

Tera's Hearty Party

SERVES 4–6

Recipe donated by Tera Prestwich.

1 head broccoli
1 head cauliflower
1 red bell pepper
1 green bell pepper
1 orange bell pepper
2 stalks celery, sliced
3 green onions
1 bag edamame (soybeans), shelled
½ cup Essential Balance oil (or oil of choice)
½ clove minced garlic
¼ cup of Bragg Liquid Aminos or 1–2 tsps. RealSalt
1 Tbs. Garlic Herb Bread Seasoning (Spice Hunter)
Zip (Spice Hunter, for garnish)

Chop the broccoli, cauliflower, bell peppers, celery, and green onions and mix together. Cook the edamame as directed and add to the mix. Then add in the oil, minced garlic, Bragg Aminos, and Garlic Herb Bread Seasoning. Toss together and garnish with Zip.

Jerusalem Salad

SERVES 4

Donated by Sue Mount.

⅓ cup tahini
2 Tbs. olive oil
1–2 cloves garlic, crushed
Juice of ½ lemon
3 Tbs. parsley
Salt or RealSalt to taste
Water
1 cucumber, diced
6 roma tomatoes, or 3 regular tomatoes, diced

Mix the first six ingredients thoroughly (through the salt) in a salad bowl; add water to thin to make a dressing. Add the cucumber and tomatoes and toss. You can let this sit for an hour to allow the flavors to meld.

Refreshing Grapefruit Salad

Serves 2–4

Donated by Kathleen C. Waite.

I like to arrange the avocado slices in this recipe like flower petals, and put the grapefruit mixture inside as the center of the flower.

1 Tbs. flax oil
1 Tbs. Bragg Liquid Aminos (or RealSalt or Herbamare
    to taste)
1–2 tsps. sesame seeds
1 tsp. Mexican seasoning (Spice Hunter) (optional)
1 grapefruit, peeled and cut into bite-sized pieces
1 cup chopped celery
1 red bell pepper, chopped or thinly sliced
1 cup grated jicama
1 handful fresh cilantro
1 avocado, peeled and sliced lengthwise
¼–½ cup soaked almonds, chopped

Combine the first four ingredients (through the Mexican spice) to make a dressing. Combine the remaining ingredients except the avocado and almonds in a bowl and toss with the dressing. Arrange on a plate with avocado slices. Top with almonds.

Steamed Beets with Greens

Serves 2–4

Donated by Kathleen Waite.

1 bunch fresh beets, with greens attached
Juice of ½ lemon

1 Tbs. flax oil
1 Tbs. Bragg Liquid Aminos (or RealSalt or Herbamare to taste)
¼–½ cup almonds, soaked and chopped (optional)

Cut the beet heads from the greens and scrub well. Trim the ends and cut into quarters or halves, depending on the size of the beet. Steam in a steaming basket on high for 10 minutes and remove from the heat. Meanwhile, wash and rinse the beet greens. Fold them over a couple of times and cut into pieces. When the beets are done, place the greens over the beets in the basket, put the lid back on, and let stand for 5 minutes to soften the greens. Meanwhile, combine the lemon juice, oil, and Bragg or salt. Put the greens and beets into a serving bowl and stir with the dressing. Top with almonds.

Romaine Peppered Salad

SERVES 6

Donated by Randy Wakefield.

1 clove minced or pressed garlic
2 tsps. cold-pressed olive oil or Essential Balance
2 tsps. minced onion
2 tsps. finely chopped tomato
1 small jalapeño pepper, seeded, and finely chopped
3 cups romaine lettuce
3 cups Belgian endive
1 red bell pepper, cut into strips
1 yellow bell pepper, cut into strips
Bragg Liquid Aminos or RealSalt to taste

Combine the garlic and oil in a small bowl; let stand for 30 minutes. Then add the minced onion, tomato, and jalapeño; stir well and set aside. Lay down whole romaine leaves to cover six salad plates. Tear the endive and remaining romaine into small pieces and layer over the top. Lay pepper strips on top. Drizzle each serving with 1½ Tbs. of the oil mixture. Sprinkle with Bragg Aminos or RealSalt to taste.

Sunshine Salad

SERVES 6–8

Donated by Frances Parkton.
Second place, pH Miracle Recipe Contest.

2 cups cooked quinoa
1 cup minced zucchini
2 cups minced broccoli
1 cup minced onion
1 red or orange bell pepper, minced
1 cup pine nuts
2 Tbs. toasted sesame oil
Salt to taste
Tomatoes, chopped, to taste
Parsley, minced, to taste
1 recipe Sunshine Dressing (see page 237)

Combine all the ingredients except the dressing in a serving bowl. Top with the dressing and serve.

Broccoli Jewels

SERVES 4–6

Donated by Brooke Peterson.

2 heads broccoli, florets chopped to 1-inch size (retain stems for
 another recipe)
1 red bell pepper, chopped (optional)
6 cloves garlic, finely chopped
Juice of 1 lemon (approximately 1 Tbs.)
¼ cup Bragg Liquid Aminos
½ cup olive oil

Mix all the ingredients together. Serve immediately, or cover and
store in a container in the refrigerator for up to 1 week.

Tabbouli (Parsley Salad)

SERVES 4–6

Donated by Jennifer Grinberg.

*Burghul is a crushed wheat that has been boiled, dried in the sun, and then
ground. You can find it in health food stores under this name, or with a
variety of spellings, such as* bulgur. *It may be found in ethnic stores under
the name* Lebanese crushed wheat. *Do not use ordinary cracked wheat.*

1 cup burghul (bulgur wheat)
6–8 bunches parsley, finely chopped (use food processor)
4–6 large tomatoes, finely chopped
¼ cup very finely chopped fresh mint leaves
2–3 tsps. dried mint
10–12 scallions, finely chopped (set aside ½ cup)
2–2½ tsps. RealSalt

1 tsp. fresh-ground pepper
¼ tsp. mixed spices: allspice, cinnamon, nutmeg, and
    cinnamon oil
¼–½ cup virgin olive oil
Juice of 3–4 lemons
Greens as garnish, preferably romaine or any firm lettuce
    leaves

Place the burghul in a large glass measuring cup, cover with warm or room-temperature water, mix with your hands, and rinse a couple of times until it's clean. Cover with water again and let sit for about 30 to 45 minutes while preparing the other ingredients. The burghul will increase in size.

Combine the finely chopped parsley, tomatoes, mint, and scallions (except for the ½ cup) in a very large mixing bowl, cover, and refrigerate. Drain the burghul by using a very fine-mesh strainer so the wheat doesn't go through. Squeeze the water out until the burghul is fairly dry. Transfer into a separate bowl and add the reserved ½ cup scallions, RealSalt, pepper, and mixed spices. Mix thoroughly. Cover and refrigerate so that all the ingredients saturate the burghul. When ready to serve, place the burghul mixture in the bottom of a very large serving bowl and place the parsley mixture on top. Toss well, being sure to bring the burghul up from the bottom and throughout the parsley mixture. Add the oil and lemon juice and toss well. Adjust the salt, pepper, and lemon to taste.

Tabbouli is served in a wide-based bowl or deep serving dish. Place lettuce leaves around the edge of the bowl as a garnish. This can be served as a meal. When served as *mezza* (hors d'oeuvres), a large spoonful is placed in the center of a lettuce leaf and wrapped into a roll to be eaten with the fingers. It can also be rolled into a fresh grape leaf (which must be picked tender and then prepared for eating by boiling in water until softened but not falling apart).

Cabbage Salad (Lebanese *Salat Malfouf*)

SERVES 4–6

Donated by Jennifer Grinberg.

1 small head green cabbage
1 small head red cabbage
2 cloves garlic
1 teaspoon RealSalt
½ cup fresh-squeezed lemon juice
½ cup virgin olive oil
Fresh-ground pepper to taste
2–3 tomatoes, diced

Remove any tough outer leaves, then cut the cabbage heads into quarters. Slice the leaves thinly and place in a large mixing bowl. Salt the leaves and set aside. Crush the garlic with the RealSalt with a mortar and pestle to form a paste. Combine with the lemon juice, olive oil, and pepper. Toss the dressing with the cabbage. Toss in the tomatoes just before serving.

Avocado Salad

SERVES 4–6

Donated by Minda Kramar.

1 head lettuce, chopped
1 cucumber, chopped
2 tomatoes, chopped
¼ red onion, thinly sliced
3 medium to large avocados, mashed
1 cup soy mayonnaise (without vinegar)
Garlic salt and pepper to taste

Toss the chopped veggies in a bowl. In a separate bowl, combine the avocados, soy mayonnaise, garlic salt, and pepper. Chill in the refrigerator. Combine all the ingredients just before serving.

Broccoli Slaw

SERVES 4

Donated by Brooke Peterson.

Stems from 2 heads broccoli (perfect if you also make Broccoli Jewels; see page 219)
½ head purple cabbage
1 medium red onion, quartered
Juice of 1 lemon or lime
¼ cup extra-virgin olive oil
¼ cup Bragg Liquid Aminos

Using an S blade in your food processor, pulse-chop the broccoli stems with the cabbage until quarter-sized. Add the onion, and pulse-chop to your desired consistency. Combine the lemon or lime juice, olive oil and Liquid Aminos, then toss the dressing with the veggies and serve. Stored in a covered container, this will last several days in the refrigerator, so prepare plenty!

Marinated Veggie-Kale Chop Salad

SERVES 8–10

Donated by Brooke Peterson.

**8–12 cups any or all of the following: curly kale, "black kale,"
    purple cabbage, carrots, onions, cauliflower, zucchini, red bell
    peppers, broccoli—your choice. Make it a rainbow!**
Juice of 1 lemon or lime
¼ cup extra-virgin olive oil
¼ cup Bragg Liquid Aminos

Using a food processor with an S blade, pulse-chop the veggies—
firmer ones first—until they are about quarter-sized. Place in a large
salad bowl. Next, pulse-chop a quarter of the kale, stems and all.
Combine the lemon or lime juice, olive oil, and Liquid Aminos,
pour over the veggies, and toss. This will keep in the refrigerator for
several days.

Alfalfa Sprout Salad

SERVES 6

3 cups alfalfa sprouts
3 cups chopped summer squash
2 red peppers, diced
2 chopped green onions
¼ cup chopped red onion

Dressing:
1 cup flaxseed oil
Juice of 1 fresh lemon or lime
1 tsp. RealSalt

1–2 tsps. seasoning blend (optional), such as Italian or Mexican (I use Spice Hunter brand)

Combine the vegetables in a large bowl. Toss with the dressing to taste.

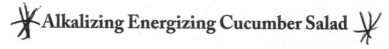

Alkalizing Energizing Cucumber Salad

SERVES 3

Cucumber is one of the most alkalizing and energizing foods that you can eat. It is considered to have a purifying effect on the digestive system and is very beneficial to the hair and skin. (For a refreshing lift, lie down with a cucumber slice over each eye for a few minutes, or rub a slice over your face after cleansing to tone and purify your skin.)

2 cups chopped cucumbers
2 Tbs. chopped parsley
1 Tbs. lemon juice
1 Tbs. flaxseed oil or olive oil
⅓ cup finely chopped peppermint

In a small serving bowl, combine the cucumbers, parsley, lemon juice, oil, and mint. Toss together. Chill for several hours or overnight. Toss again before serving.

Colorful Cabbage

SERVES 4

Cabbage is considered one of the most powerful therapeutic foods in the world. Many studies have linked eating cabbage with a reduction of

*cancer, especially colon cancer. Also, cabbage juice has been proven to help
heal stomach ulcers and prevent stomach cancer.*

2 cups red cabbage, thinly sliced
2 cups green cabbage, thinly sliced
1 carrot, grated
1 red pepper, slivered
1 yellow pepper, slivered
1 green pepper, slivered
1 orange pepper, slivered
4 Tbs. chopped scallions
4 Tbs. minced parsley
¼ cup lemon juice
3 Tbs. water
1 Tbs. oil (extra-virgin olive, flaxseed, or Udo's Choice)
1–2 tsps. dried red chili pepper
Dash of Bragg Liquid Aminos

In a bowl, combine all the ingredients. Toss thoroughly and let the
flavors mix for at least half an hour before serving.

Spinach Salad

SERVES 2–3

1 head spinach
½ cup cauliflower, cut in small pieces
2 stalks celery, chopped
6 radishes, chopped
2 shallots (or 1 small red onion), chopped
½ cup chopped basil
2 red peppers, chopped
4 Tbs. pine nuts

In a large bowl, combine all the ingredients and toss well. Top with Essential Dressing (see page 245).

DRESSINGS, DIPS, AND SAUCES

The sauce is often the tastiest part of a meal. Veggies always taste more exciting dressed with herbs, seasonings, and spices. It's also a way to include creamy textures in your dishes and enrich them with healthy and essential fats.

Almond Chili Sauce

SERVES 2–4

Donated by Roxy Boelz.
Third place, pH Miracle Recipe Contest.

½ cup raw almond butter
1 Tbs. grated fresh ginger
2 Tbs. lemon juice
1 clove garlic
1 Tbs. Bragg Liquid Aminos
1 chili, such as serrano
¼ cup water

Blend all the ingredients together in a blender till smooth. Add the water gradually, until you get the consistency you desire.

Mock Sour Cream

SERVES 2–4

Donated by Roxy Boelz.
Third place, pH Miracle Recipe Contest.

¾ cup coconut meat
⅓ cup Brazil nuts (soaked overnight)
3 Tbs. olive oil
2 Tbs. lemon juice
1 Tbs. water
½ tsp. RealSalt

Blend all the ingredients until smooth. Add the water gradually to get the consistency you want.

Flaxseed Oil and Lemon Dressing

SERVES 2–4

Donated by Roxy Boelz.
Third place, pH Miracle Recipe Contest.

⅓ bunch fresh basil (or 1–2 tsps. dried)
2 cloves garlic
½ cup lemon juice
¼ cup flaxseed oil or Udo's Blend
¼ cup water
¼ cup olive oil

Combine the basil and garlic in a blender. Add the rest of the ingredients and blend to your desired consistency.

Sunny Spread

SERVES 2–4

Donated by Roxy Boelz.
Third place, pH Miracle Recipe Contest.

1 cup sunflower seeds (soaked for 6 hours or overnight)
1 cup almonds (soaked for 6 hours or overnight)
2 Tbs. lemon juice
½ cup fresh herbs of choice (parsley, basil, cilantro, etc.)
1 Tbs. dulse flakes

Process the sunflower seeds and almonds in a food processor. Add the remaining ingredients except the dulse flakes and stir well. Sprinkle on the dulse flakes.

Variations: For garlic flavor, add chopped garlic to the lemon juice and herbs, then combine with the sunflower/almond mixture. Or use 1 tsp. kelp instead of dulse flakes, adding the kelp in the food processor with the rest of the ingredients.

Almond Butter Dressing

SERVES 2–4

Donated by Debra Jenkins. First place, pH Miracle Recipe Contest, Transitional Recipes Category.

1–2 Tbs. almond butter
¼ lb. soft or silken tofu
1 fresh clove garlic
2–4 Tbs. oil (Udo's Blend, Essential Balance blend, or olive oil)
Juice of 1 lime
½–1 Tbs. Bragg Liquid Aminos

1 tsp. Spice Hunter Mesquite Seasoning
½ tsp. onion powder

Blend all the ingredients together.

Tofu Hummus

SERVES 2–3

Donated by Debra Jenkins.
First place, pH Miracle Recipe Contest,
Transitional Recipes Category.

8 oz. tofu
½ cup raw tahini
Juice of ½ lemon
1 tsp. cumin
2–3 sun-dried peppers or tomatoes
1 clove garlic
½ tsp. RealSalt

Blend all the ingredients together.

Almond Gravy

SERVES 2–3

Donated by Debra Jenkins.
First place, pH Miracle Recipe Contest,
Transitional Recipes Category.

This is good over buckwheat, rice, veggie burgers, vegetables, salmon, and more.

2 cups water
½ cup almonds (soaked and blanched, if preferred)
2 Tbs. arrowroot powder
2 tsp. onion powder
2 Tbs. grape seed oil
½ tsp. RealSalt

Blend all the ingredients together. Then warm over high heat, stirring constantly until thickened, about 3 minutes.

Tofu "Whipped Cream"

SERVES 2–4

Donated by Debra Jenkins.
First place, pH Miracle Recipe Contest,
Transitional Recipes Category.

Use this as a topping in place of whipped cream, over warmed grains or dessert selections such as Pumpkin Crème Pie (page 281) or Avocado Coconut Key Lime Pie (page 283), also by Debra.

8 oz. silken tofu
2 tsps. Frontier nonalcoholic vanilla extract

⅛ tsp. stevia
1 Tbs. lemon juice
Water or almond milk
1½ tsps. psyllium or agar flakes (optional)

Drain the tofu thoroughly. Combine the tofu, vanilla, stevia, and lemon juice in a food processor and blend. Add water or almond milk as needed to create a smooth consistency (this should take only a few tablespoons). To make the "whipped cream" stiffer, add psyllium or agar. Refrigerate until chilled.

Variation: Flavor with cinnamon.

Nutty Crème Topping

SERVES 1–2

Donated by Debra Jenkins.
First place, pH Miracle Recipe Contest,
Transitional Recipes Category.

½ cup almonds
⅓ cup boiling water
½ tsp. lemon juice
Stevia

In a blender or coffee grinder, grind the almonds to a fine powder. Add the water and juice, then add stevia to taste (about 2 to 3 drops of liquid, or 1 pkg.). Blend on high till smooth and creamy. Chill for an hour or two.

Variation: Flavor with cinnamon, or almond or maple flavoring (be sure to get the kind without alcohol).

Almond Avocado Dressing

SERVES 2–4

Donated by Debra Jenkins.
First place, pH Miracle Recipe Contest,
Transitional Recipes Category.

2 Tbs. raw almond butter
1 clove garlic
½ medium avocado
1 Tbs. fresh lemon juice
1 Tbs. Bragg Liquid Aminos
3 Tbs. Essential Balance oil blend
3 Tbs. Udo's Blend (or favorite olive oil)
Dash of garlic powder
½ tsp. onion powder
½ tsp. Frontier Spice Fajita Seasonings

Blend all the ingredients in a blender until smooth and creamy.
Chill.

Variation: Add 3 or 4 sun-dried tomatoes.

Avocado Grapefruit Dressing

SERVES 1–2

Donated by Debra Jenkins.
First place, pH Miracle Recipe Contest,
Transitional Recipes Category.

1 large avocado
Juice of 1 small or ½ large grapefruit
Stevia (optional)

Blend the avocado and juice in a blender, then add stevia to balance the tang, if desired.

⚡ Chips and Salsa ⚡

SERVES 4

Donated by Kelly Anclien.
First place, pH Miracle Recipe Contest,
Alkalizing Recipes Category.

This recipe is great served as part of Kelly's other recipe, Fiesta Tacos El Alkalarian (see page 249).

Chips:
Sprouted-wheat tortillas
Olive oil
Garlic pepper
Fajita seasoning
RealSalt

Salsa:
2 large tomatoes
5 Tbs. diced purple or red onion
1½ jalapeño peppers, seeded and chopped (mild salsa)
3 tsps. chopped fresh cilantro
2 garlic cloves, minced
1 tsp. fresh lemon juice
RealSalt to taste
½ tsp. pepper
2 sun-dried tomatoes (optional)

Preheat the oven to 350 degrees. Rub oil onto both sides of each tortilla, and sprinkle one side with spices (those above, or any combination you dream up). Use a pizza cutter to slice each tortilla into eight triangles. Bake on a cookie sheet for 13 minutes, or until crispy.

Meanwhile, make the salsa by placing the remaining ingredients into a food processor and blending to your desired consistency. Use the sun-dried tomatoes if desired to sweeten and thicken the salsa.

Decadent Dill Spread

SERVES 4

Donated by Eric Prouty.
Second place, pH Miracle Recipe Contest,
Alkalizing Recipes Category.

Serve this spread on cucumber slices, celery stalks, sushi nori paper (for veggie rolls), flax crackers, or sprouted tortillas (for veggie wraps).

2 cups soaked sunflower seeds
3 cloves garlic
⅓ onion
2 Tbs. olive oil
1 Tbs. Bragg Liquid Aminos (or ½–1 tsp. RealSalt)
1 tsp. dill

Use a Green Star/Green Life or Champion juicer with a plug attachment for nut butters. Add the seeds, garlic, and onion. Mix with the remaining ingredients in a bowl.

Tomata Tostada Basilicious

SERVES 8–10

Donated by Dianne Ellsworth.

Use your favorite premade tortillas for this recipe—or make your own. Dianne likes to tweak the Shelley's Super Tortillas recipe found in The pH Miracle *by adding about 20 sun-dried tomatoes, an additional 2 to 4 basil leaves, a roasted green chili (peeled and seeded) and reducing the amount of coconut milk or water to achieve the correct consistency for dough.*

2–3 Tbs. olive oil
Juice of 1 lime
1–2 garlic cloves, minced
⅛–¼ cup tahini (raw)
1 jar (17 oz.) garbanzo beans, drained (save water)
20–22 sun-dried tomatoes packed in olive oil
8–10 basil leaves (plus additional for garnish)
RealSalt, to taste
½–1 tsp. Garlic Herb Bread Seasoning (Spice Hunter)
½–1 tsp. cumin
Zip (Spice Hunter), to taste
2–6 tortillas
1–2 tomatoes, sliced
1–2 cups guacamole

In a food processor, process the oil, lime juice, garlic, and tahini until smooth. Add the beans, sun-dried tomatoes, and seasonings and process until creamy. You may need to thin with extra water (from the beans) to your desired consistency. Spread the hummus on tortillas, add a layer of tomato slices and a layer of guacamole, and garnish with sliced basil leaves.

Texas-Style Guacamole

SERVES 2

Donated by Amy Efeney.

Serve chilled or at room temperature, with veggies or tortilla chips (try Shelley's homemade tortilla chips with Mexican Seasoning in The pH Miracle*). This is a great after-work pick-me-up snack.*

2 large avocados
1 whole jalapeño pepper (more or less)
½ habanero pepper (or not—they're really hot!)
¼ cup onion
¼ cup roasted tomatoes (or fresh)
1 tsp. fresh lemon juice
1 shot garlic powder
1 shot RealSalt
1–2 shots fresh-ground pepper

Mash all the ingredients together with a fork for chunky guacamole, or use a blender (a new one might have a "salsa" setting) or food processor for smoother texture.

Avocado Salad Dressing

SERVES 4–6

Donated by Gerry Johnson.

Delicious over a garden salad.

2 ripe avocados, peeled
1 cup freshly juiced celery juice
Seasonings (optional)

Mix the avocados and juice together in a blender, adjusting the amount of juice to achieve your desired consistency. Add whatever seasonings appeal to you—or enjoy as is.

Sunshine Dressing

Serves 6–8

Donated by Frances Parkton.
Second place, pH Miracle Recipe Contest.

This is a great versatile dressing, dip, or sauce—somewhat like an all-around hollandaise sauce that you could use for almost any dish. Great over tacos or burritos, too!

2 cups minced cucumber
2 sun-dried tomatoes
1 cup minced onions
4 jalapeños, minced
1 cup minced green bell pepper
½ cup olive oil
½ cup avocado oil
¼ cup veganaise (make sure it doesn't have vinegar)
2 tsps. Mexican Seasoning
Juice of 2 limes
2 tsps. Herbamare
½ tsp. cayenne pepper
2 tsps. fresh garlic

Put all the ingredients into a Vita-Mix or blender and blend to make a salad dressing. Adjust the seasonings to taste.

Variation: Add 1 cup on up to 4 pts. of cherry tomatoes for a wonderful gazpacho.

Rustic Guacamole

SERVES 4–6

Donated by Maraline Krey.
Second place, pH Miracle Recipe Contest,
Transitional Recipes Category.

This guacamole can be served as a side dish or as a main-course salad over baby spinach drenched in lime juice and avocado or olive oil. For a great salsa to use over fish, add a cut-up grapefruit.

4 Haas avocados, diced into ½- to ¾-inch cubes
½ bunch cilantro, cut up (use kitchen scissors)
1 extra-large or 2–3 small tomatoes, diced
¼ onion, chopped
Juice of 2–3 limes
½ tsp. RealSalt
½–1 tsp. Zip (Spice Hunter) or hot sauce (optional)

Combine all the ingredients in a large bowl and toss as you would a salad. Keeps in the refrigerator for 2 days.

Pesto Dressing/Sauce

SERVES 4

Serve cold over salad or veggies or legumes.

½ jar Garlic Galore Pesto (Rising Sun Farms brand has no dairy)
½ cup olive oil (cold-pressed virgin)
2–3 sun-dried tomatoes
1 tsp. Garlic Herb Bread Seasoning (Spice Hunter)
½ cup raw macadamia nuts
Water to desired consistency

Put all the ingredients into a food processor and process until smooth, adding water to your desired consistency.

Fresh Garlic-Herb Dressing

SERVES 4

¾ cup Essential Balance oil, a blend of organic, flax, pumpkin, and sunflower oils (Omega Nutrition)
Juice of 1 large lime
1 tsp. Italian Pizza Seasoning (Spice Hunter)
2–3 cloves fresh garlic, minced
½ tsp. onion salt (RealSalt puts out a nice blend)
½ tsp. Vegetable Rub (Spice Hunter)
¼ tsp. fresh-minced rosemary
¼ tsp. Heat Wave Seasoning (a very hot spice from the Cape Herb and Spice Company)

Blend all the ingredients in a food processor or blender until well blended.

RANCHadamia Super Sauce

SERVES 6–8

This is a great way to get off dairy ranch salad dressing. It is also great as a dip for raw veggies, or as a spread in wraps. Macadamias are rich in unsaturated fats and contain calcium, magnesium, and many of the amino acids that make complete proteins.

2 cups fresh raw macadamia nuts
Juice of 1 lemon

2–6 tsps. Litehouse Salad Herbs seasoning (a freeze-dried combination of parsley, shallots, chives, onions, and garlic)
6–9 sun-dried tomatoes
1½ tsps. Spice Hunter Cafe Solé Lemon Pepper (a blend of
lemon, pepper, onion, and sea salt)
2 squirts Bragg Liquid Aminos
Water

With the food processor running (using an S blade), add all the
ingredients except the water through the top chute. Start with 2 tsps.
of seasoning, then taste and adjust the amount. Mix well and then
slowly pour in a large glass of water until you reach your desired consistency. Process until very creamy.

Three-Citrus Dressing

SERVES 6–8 (APPROXIMATELY 2 CUPS)

*This is a nice thick dressing with a sweet-and-sour taste . . . very zingy!
It is good when you are phasing out Thousand Island and other sweet
dressings.*

Juice of ½ large pink grapefruit
Juice of 1 lime
Juice of 1 lemon
½ tsp. chicory root powder (Nature's Taste by Amazon), or 6–10
drops liquid stevia extract, or 1–2 pkgs. powdered stevia
1 tsp. hot mustard powder
4 Tbs. dried onion
2 tsps. garlic powder
2 tsps. dried basil
¼ tsp. dried rosemary
½ tsp. RealSalt
Pinch of Zip or to taste

1½ cups Essential Balance oil (Arrowhead Mills or Omega Nutrition brand) or other healthy oil
1 heaping Tbs. flaxseeds

Put all but the last two ingredients into a food processor or blender and blend well. With the machine still running, add the oil, then the flaxseeds, and let machine run until all the ingredients are well emulsified.

Citrus, Flax, and Poppy Seed Dressing

SERVES 4

Donated by Derry Bresee.

½ cup carrot juice
½ cup freshly squeezed citrus juice (juice of 2 lemons or ½ grapefruit)
½ tsp. dry mustard powder
2 Tbs. minced dry onion
1 tsp. flaxseeds (optional)
1 tsp. minced fresh garlic
1 tsp. basil
½ tsp. RealSalt
1 Tbs. poppy seeds
1 cup flaxseed oil

Combine all but the last two ingredients in a blender and blend, using the flaxseeds if you want a thicker dressing. Add the poppy seeds and pulse briefly. With the blender on low, slowly pour the oil in until the dressing is emulsified and thickened.

Flaxseed Oil Dressing

SERVES 2–4

Donated by Derry Bresee.

Juice of 1 lemon or lime (about ¼ cup)
½ tsp. onion powder
½ tsp. garlic powder
½ tsp. salt
½ tsp. chopped dried basil
1 Tbs. flaxseeds (optional—use if you want to thicken enough that
    it spreads like mayonnaise)
½ cup flaxseed oil (or twice as much as the juice; shake the bottle
    well before pouring)

Blend all the ingredients in a blender. Serve immediately, or refrigerate until use.

Variation: Use your favorite herbs or spices instead of the seasonings listed here.

Garlic French Dressing

SERVES 8

Donated by Myra Marvez.

½ cup dried tomato
1 whole lemon
3 large cloves garlic
1 tsp. RealSalt
1 tsp. paprika
½ tsp. cayenne pepper

1–2 pkgs. stevia
2 cups or more water

Blend all the ingredients together in a Vita-Mix, adding up to 20 oz. of water to your desired consistency. This should be thick and creamy.

Almonnaise

SERVES 2–4

Donated by Myra Marvez.

This is good in wraps, as a dip for veggies, or as a base for salad dressings.

½ cup raw almonds
2 scoops Super Soy Powder
2 cloves garlic
1 tsp. RealSalt
1 whole lemon, peeled
1–1½ cups light oil

Bring 2 cups water to a vigorous boil. Put the almonds in for about 30 seconds, then remove promptly into a strainer. Their skins should come off easily, but if they don't, repeat this procedure. Place the skinless almonds in a food processor with the soy powder, garlic, salt, and lemon. Run the processor and very slowly add the oil. Continue processing until a thick, creamy consistency is obtained. Almonnaise keeps in the fridge for a week.

Spinach Artichoke Dip

SERVES 8–10

Donated by Brooke Peterson.

Here's a close approximation of that old party favorite, but without any dairy.

2 cups almonds, soaked for 8 hours, then rinsed
2–3 cloves garlic or 6 slightly roasted garlic cloves and 2 tsps. garlic powder
1 can (14 oz.) quartered artichoke hearts packed in water
Up to ½ cup green drink, if needed
Juice of 1 lemon or lime (approximately 1 Tbs.)
2 Tbs. olive oil
1 Tbs. Bragg Liquid Aminos or ½ tsp. RealSalt (if using the roasted garlic)
1 scoop green powder (optional)
1 scoop soy sprouts powder (optional)
8 cups spinach

Using an S blade in your food processor, blend the almonds with garlic, the liquid from the can of artichokes (approximately ½ cup), and a quarter of the can of artichokes. Let the food processor run until the almonds have completely broken up and the mixture has become smooth. Add green drink if needed. Add the lemon juice, olive oil, and Liquid Aminos or RealSalt (if using), plus the green powder and the sprouted soy powder if you want that nutritional boost. Taste and adjust the garlic, lemon, and salt as desired. Add spinach by handfuls and process, scraping down the sides frequently. When the spinach is incorporated, pulse-chop the remaining artichokes into the mixture until your desired consistency is achieved. (I like it chunky.) Serve in three hollowed-out red, yellow, or orange bell peppers, displayed on a beautiful bed of greens (kale holds up nicely), with your choice of veggies for dipping, such as cucumber, celery, carrot, and zucchini.

Soy Cucumber Dressing

SERVES 4

A subtle, refreshing dressing.

2–3 tsps. carrot juice
1 large cucumber (I prefer peeled and seeded)
½ red bell pepper
½ small onion
1 cup soy milk
1 tsp. dried basil (or 2 tsps. fresh)
1 Tbs. Bragg Liquid Aminos or RealSalt, to taste

Blend all the ingredients in a food processor or blender until smooth.

Essential Dressing

SERVES 4–6

1 cup preferred oil (Udo's, Essential Balance, olive, flaxseed, or grape seed)
¼ cup Bragg Liquid Aminos or 1 tsp. RealSalt (adjust to taste)
Juice of 1 fresh lemon
½–1 tsp. of any seasoning you prefer, such as Italian, Mexican (Spice Hunter), pesto, garlic powder, onion powder, parsley, basil, or oregano

Combine all the ingredients in a food processor and mix well—or simply place in a salad dressing jar and shake to mix well. Chill and serve.

Lime Ginger Sauce

SERVES 4–6

¼ cup lime juice
¼ cup oil (flaxseed, olive, or Udo's Choice)
1 Tbs. Bragg Liquid Aminos
¼ cup water
1 Tbs. fresh mint
1 Tbs. fresh cilantro
1 tsp. minced gingerroot
¼ tsp. dried red chili pepper
2–3 tsps. fresh jicama or carrot juice
1 tsp. RealSalt, to taste
Dash of Zip (Spice Hunter)

In a blender or food processor, combine all the ingredients and blend well.

ENTRÉES/SIDE DISHES

The following dishes range from casual to gourmet, and offer some of the best sources of animal protein, good fats, and complementary seasonings. Whether they are entrées or side dishes depends on the balance you need to strike: Keep at least a 70:30 ratio on your plate, with the majority of your meal being raw veggies.

Coconut and Macadamia Nut Crested Salmon

SERVES 6

This is a wonderfully sweet Hawaiian rendition of salmon I use for special occasions. It always gets rave reviews at pH Miracle retreats!

3 cups dehydrated unsweetened coconut flakes
3 cups raw macadamia nuts
1 tsp. RealSalt
2 tsps. Garlic Herb Bread Seasoning (Spice Hunter)
Juice of 3 limes
1 can coconut milk (Thai brand)
6 salmon fillets sliced very thin (½ inch)
Grape seed oil, for frying

Combine the coconut flakes, macadamias, salt, and seasoning in a food processor. Pulse-chop to mix, then let the machine run until the mixture is finely ground and crumbly. Combine the lime juice and coconut milk. Dip the fillets into the liquid, then into the coconut mixture to coat heavily. Press and pat the coating into the fish. In an electric skillet on medium heat, fry for 4 to 6 minutes, or until golden brown. Flip just once and fry on the other side until golden. If the fish is not done in the center, place the lid over the skillet and steam until done. Lift each fillet onto a serving platter with a spatula, taking care lest the coating crumble off. Serve immediately.

Asparagus with Garlic-Lemon Sauce

SERVES 1–2

Donated by Roxy Boelz.
Third place, pH Miracle Recipe Contest,
Alkalizing Recipes Category.

2 cups asparagus, steamed
⅓ cup fresh lemon juice
3 Tbs. ground golden flaxseeds
1 chopped garlic clove

Lightly steam the asparagus. Add the lemon juice, ground flaxseed, and garlic, and stir. Serve warm or cold.

Tomato Asparagus Ratatouille

SERVES 2–4

Donated by Debra Jenkins.
First place, pH Miracle Recipe Contest,
Transitional Recipes Category.

Serve on its own or over wild rice, buckwheat, or spelt noodles. Makes a great alkaline anytime meal . . . even breakfast!

1 medium eggplant, peeled and cubed
1 cup chopped asparagus
½ cup chopped green beans
1 chopped onion
1 clove garlic, minced or grated
1 small zucchini, sliced
3–4 fresh tomatoes
¼ tsp. cayenne pepper
½ tsp. garlic powder
1 tsp. onion powder
1–2 tsps. Spice Hunter Mesquite Seasoning
1–2 cups fresh spinach (optional)
¼ cup olive oil (use garlic- or rosemary-flavored for extra zip)
RealSalt and /or Bragg Liquid Aminos to taste

Lightly sauté all the vegetables except the spinach in water in a skillet for 2 to 4 minutes. Stir in the seasonings. Add the spinach (if using) and stir for 30 seconds more. Remove from the heat, pour olive oil over it all, and sprinkle with Bragg Aminos. Serve immediately.

Variation: Add a few white beans or tofu.

Fiesta Tacos El Alkalarian

SERVES 4–6

Donated by Kelly Anclien.
First place, pH Miracle Recipe Contest,
Transitional Recipes Category.

The tacos:
2 sprouted-wheat tortillas
Olive oil
Spice Hunter Garlic Pepper
Spice Hunter Fajita Seasoning
RealSalt

The salsa:
2 large tomatoes, peeled and seeded, or 2 sun-dried tomatoes
5 Tbs. diced purple or red onion
1½ tsps. jalapeño pepper, seeded (mild salsa)
3 tsps. fresh cilantro
2 garlic cloves, minced
1 tsp. fresh lemon juice
½ tsp. ground pepper

The guacamole:
2 avocados, mashed with a fork
½ tsp. Spice Hunter Mesquite Seasoning
½ tsp. Spice Hunter Fajita Seasoning
¼ tsp. RealSalt

Putting it all together:
1 can (16 oz.) refried beans
1–2 red bell peppers, sliced into strips
Mixed greens to fill a salad bowl (about 1 medium bag, 16–24 oz.)

Line the bottom oven rack with tinfoil. Preheat the oven to 350
degrees. Rub olive oil onto both sides of each tortilla, and sprinkle
one side with Garlic Pepper, Fajita Seasoning, and salt. Hang each

tortilla over two bars of the upper oven rack to form the shape of tacos. (Any dripping oil will land on the tinfoil.) Bake for 13 minutes, or until crisp.

Meanwhile, make the salsa by blending the tomatoes, onion, jalapeño, cilantro, garlic, lemon juice, and ground pepper in a food processor to your desired consistency. Use sun-dried tomatoes if you like a sweeter, thicker salsa. Add RealSalt to taste.

Make the guacamole by stirring together the avocado with the Mesquite and Fajita Seasonings and RealSalt. Assemble Fiesta Tacos with layers of refried beans, salsa, guacamole, red peppers, and mixed greens.

Roasted Veggie Pizzas

SERVES 8–10

I developed this recipe by basically unwrapping Shelley's Super Wraps (from The pH Miracle*), roasting the veggies, and crisping the tortillas. These are by far the favorite dinner at pH Miracle retreats. Feel free to add to or change the veggies you use in any way that appeals to you. Eggplant, bok choy, celery, and snow peas, anyone?*

3 red bell peppers
2–3 orange bell peppers
1–2 green bell peppers
2 sweet onions (I use yellow)
20–30 whole cloves garlic
4 yellow crookneck squash
3 zucchinis
2 large heads broccoli, cut into florets
1–2 heads cauliflower, chopped
Grape seed oil
3 avocados, sliced

1 pkg. (6–8) sprouted-wheat tortillas
2 cups hummus or 1 recipe Yummus Hummus from *The pH Miracle*
2 cups nondairy pesto or 1 recipe Spring's Pesto from *The pH Miracle*
1 tube (8–12 oz.) sun-dried tomato paste (or make your own by
    whirling 12–15 sun-dried tomatoes in a food processor)
1 bag (1 lb.) pine nuts or slivered almonds (optional)

Preheat the broiler. Cut the veggies, except the avocados, into bite-sized chunks. Place on cookie sheets and lightly sprinkle with grape seed oil. Broil until lightly browned on the edges, about 15 minutes. Meanwhile, spread a thick layer of hummus and pesto on each tortilla. Top with generous amounts of roasted veggies, and top with avocado and some squirts of sun-dried tomato paste. Sprinkle with nuts if desired. Place under the broiler until the tortillas have crisped and the veggies are sizzling hot, and serve immediately.

Wild Fajita Verde with Ensalada Mexico

SERVES 2–3

Donated by Lory Fabbi.

½ red bell pepper, sliced in long, ¼-inch-wide strips
½ green bell pepper, sliced in long, ¼-inch-wide strips
2 Tbs. roasted green chilis, diced
½ small white or yellow onion, thinly sliced
2–3 sprouted-wheat tortillas or fresh homemade spelt tortillas (or
    use 1 large lettuce leaf in place of each tortilla)
15 fresh cilantro leaves, rolled between fingers to crush
Lime juice to taste
½ avocado, sliced
½ cup cooked kashi pilaf (whole grains) or brown rice
Salsa verde (no vinegar; I use Herdez brand)
Dash of Bragg Liquid Aminos (optional)

Sauté the peppers in a small nonstick pan wiped sparingly with oil, or grill them on a Foreman-type grill, 3 to 4 minutes, until tender but still crunchy. Cook the onion slices the same way until translucent. Warm the tortillas in a pan, then remove and fill them with peppers and onions. Top with cilantro, lime juice, avocado, rice or kashi, salsa verde, and Liquid Aminos, if desired. Serve with Ensalada Mexico (below).

Ensalada Mexico

The perfect complement to Wild Fajita Verde. Or, to make it a main course on its own, serve it with homemade tortilla chips and a dip made of refried beans, salsa, lime juice, and chopped onion, thinned slightly with water.

½ sliced red onion
1 chopped bell pepper
½ cup chopped jicama
2–3 radishes, sliced
1 chopped ripe tomato
½ avocado, chopped
½ cup black or kidney beans (optional)
Salsa (no vinegar)

Mix all the ingredients except the salsa together, and top with your favorite fresh salsa.

Variation: Mix 1 or 2 Tbs. Vegannaise with ½ cup salsa in a food processor or blender for a creamier dressing. Or, to boost the spiciness, add ¼ jalapeño, peeled, seeded, and chopped. (*Warning:* Wash your hands immediately after handling jalapeños to remove any hot pepper oil, which can otherwise really sting.)

pH Pizza Delight

SERVES 1–2

Donated by David Martini.

So fast, tasty, and alkaline, you can enjoy this anytime.

1 sprouted-wheat tortilla (large burrito size)
Hummus
Bell peppers in assorted colors
Fresh cucumbers
Fresh spinach
Tofu
Sun-dried tomatoes packed in olive oil
Spice Hunter seasoning of your choice

Spread the hummus evenly on the tortilla. Cut the toppings into slices. (Roll the spinach leaves up.) Place the veggies on the hummus in whatever design or pattern you like. Sprinkle with your favorite Spice Hunter seasoning. Slice into wedges and enjoy!

China Moon Vegetable Pasta with Coconut Lotus Sauce

SERVES 6–8

Donated by Lisa El-Kerdi.
Best in Show, pH Miracle Recipe Contest.

This colorful and flavorful dish is highly adaptable. Feel free to add vegetables of your choice, modify according to season, and adjust quantities to suit the number of friends you are serving.

1 large or 2 small spaghetti squash
1 bunch scallions, cut into 2-inch diagonals
1 carrot, thinly sliced
1–2 cups broccoli florets
½ lb. asparagus, cut into 2-inch diagonals
1 red bell pepper, sliced
2 yellow squash, sliced
1 zucchini, sliced
4–6 tiny bok choy, leaves separated, or ½ stalk large bok choy, sliced
½ lb. snow peas
1–1½ cups Coconut Lotus Sauce (recipe follows)
Shredded unsweetened coconut
Black sesame seeds

Cover the lower oven rack with aluminum foil to catch any drippings. Preheat the oven to 375 to 400 degrees. Make a 1-inch slit in top of the spaghetti squash. Bake on the upper oven rack for 30 to 50 minutes, until the squash gives to gentle pressure but is not mushy. Bring water to a boil in the bottom of a large pot with a steamer tray, then reduce to a simmer. Place the vegetables in the steamer starting with the scallions and carrot and continuing in the order listed above. Cover and steam gently for 3 to 5 minutes, then turn off the heat. The stored heat will continue to cook the vegetables. Be careful not to let them get overdone!

Cut the spaghetti squash in half and scoop the seeds out of the center. Run a fork lengthwise along the inside of the squash to form "spaghetti," and scoop gently onto plates or into shallow bowls. When the veggies are done, remove the steamer tray from the pot. (Save the broth for a soup base!) Return the vegetables to the pot, toss gently with the desired amount of sauce, and spoon on top of the squash. Garnish with coconut and sesame seeds.

Coconut Lotus Sauce

*Besides making China Moon Vegetable Pasta, you can use this versatile
sauce on a stir-fry or as a dressing or dip.*

2-inch piece gingerroot, peeled and sliced
2 large cloves garlic
½ tsp. crushed red pepper flakes (adjust to desired heat)
½ cup Bragg Liquid Aminos (or more to taste)
2 Tbs. toasted sesame oil
2 Tbs. flaxseed oil
1 cup unsweetened coconut milk (I prefer Thai Kitchen), or more
    if desired
¼ cup water, carrot juice, or vegetable broth (optional)
RealSalt to taste

Blend the first three ingredients in a food processor or Vita-Mix.
Add the Bragg and blend until smooth. Pour into a jar, add the oils,
coconut milk, and water, and shake. Thin with more water, carrot
juice, or vegetable broth if desired. Add salt to taste. Store in the
refrigerator.

Variations: For Thai Lotus Sauce, add the juice of 1 lime, 2 Tbs.
fresh or 1 tsp. dried lemongrass, 1 tsp. fresh or ½ tsp. dried basil, and
chopped fresh cilantro if desired.

For Basic Lotus Sauce, omit the coconut milk and increase the
flaxseed oil to ¼ to ⅓ cup.

For Lotus Dressing, to ½ cup of Basic Lotus Sauce add ¼ cup lime
juice, 1½ cups flaxseed or untoasted sesame oil, ½ carrot (optional),
and ½ sweet onion (optional). Blend until smooth.

For Indonesian Dipping Sauce, to ¾ cup Basic Lotus Sauce
add 1 cup almond butter, ¼ tsp. crushed red pepper (or to taste),
and ½ to 1 cup unsweetened coconut milk to reach your desired consistency.

North African Bean Stew

SERVES 4–6

Donated by Lisa El-Kerdi.
Best in Show, pH Miracle Recipe Contest.

This rich and exotic stew is sure to spice up any gathering. Serve with Moroccan Mint Salad, page 209.

1½ cups uncooked seven-bean and barley mix (or any mix of dried
    beans), soaked overnight, rinsed, and drained
1 bay leaf
⅛ tsp. cinnamon
4 cloves garlic
2 onions, quartered
4 carrots, cut into chunks
4 stalks celery, cut into chunks
1 large or 2 small eggplant
½ tsp. turmeric
1 tsp. coriander
1 tsp. cumin
½ tsp. cardamom
⅛ tsp. black pepper
⅛ tsp. cayenne
3–4 cloves garlic, pressed
1 red bell pepper
1 yellow bell pepper
2–3 yellow squash
2–3 zucchinis
4 chopped tomatoes or 1 box Pomì chopped tomatoes
1 tsp. RealSalt, plus more for eggplant
Olive oil

Cover the beans with 2½ inches of water in a large pot and add the bay leaf and cinnamon. Bring to a boil and skim off the foam.

Reduce the heat to low and simmer, covered, for 30 minutes. Chop the garlic, onions, carrots, and celery in a food processor. Add to the beans after 30 minutes of cooking. Simmer until the beans are cooked, 1 to 1½ hours. Cube and generously salt the eggplant. Let sit for 30 to 60 minutes.

While the eggplant is salting, sauté the spices in olive oil. Add to the beans. Chop the peppers. Rinse the eggplant and squeeze out the juices. Add the eggplant and peppers to the beans. Simmer for 30 minutes. Cut the squash in half lengthwise and slice. Add to the stew. Simmer for 10 minutes. Add the tomatoes and salt to the stew, and simmer for another 10 minutes. Adjust the salt to taste. Ladle into deep bowls and top each serving with 1 Tbs. olive oil (or to taste).

Spicy Kale Slaw

SERVES 4

Donated by Deborah Johnson.
Second place in pH Miracle Recipe Contest,
Alkalizing Recipes Category.

1 ripe avocado, seeded and peeled
2 cups peeled and cubed jicama
Juice of 1 lime
1 scoop soy sprouts powder
1 Tbs. Udo's Choice oil
½ tsp. RealSalt to taste
1 carrot, washed and cut into 1-inch pieces
3 kale spines, cut into 1-inch pieces
1–1½ jalapeño peppers (depending on how hot you like your food)
1 tomatillo, peeled and quartered
½ tsp. mustard seeds
3 kale leaves, torn into large pieces

Place the first six ingredients (through the salt) in a food processor or Vita-Mix and blend until smooth. Stop the machine. While the ingredients are still in the processing bowl, add the remaining ingredients in the order given. Process just until all ingredients are chopped to your desired consistency. If you're using a processor, pulse and scrape the bowl. With a Vita-Mix, use a tamping tool, and do not overprocess. This is a good lunch for one or a great side dish for two.

Fantastic Kale

SERVES 4

Donated by Wendy J. Pauluk.

Kale is a calcium-rich, chewy, dark green leafy vegetable. It is good juiced or in the raw salad below.

1 bunch kale
1 small red onion
1 red bell pepper
¼ cup olive oil
Juice of 1 lemon
Zip seasoning (Spice Hunter)

Tear the kale into bite-sized pieces; do not use the center stems. Slice the red onion and red bell pepper into thin strips and add to the kale. Add the olive oil and toss. (You can add more or less depending on the salad's size.) Refrigerate overnight in a covered bowl. Add the lemon juice and Zip seasoning to taste before serving.

Super Stuffed Tomatoes

SERVES 2–4

Donated by Frances Fujii.

This makes a beautiful presentation.

1 cup (dry) black beans
Vegetable seasoning salt (I like Herbamare)
2 cups (uncooked) wild rice (or use half brown and half wild rice)
1 medium onion, diced
4 cloves garlic, diced
Macadamia oil
2 lbs. Swiss chard, coarsely chopped (or substitute kale, spinach,
    beet greens, or other preferred leafy green vegetable)
Bragg Liquid Aminos
2 pkgs. firm tofu
6 medium-sized tomatoes
Udo's Choice oil or olive oil

Soak the black beans overnight. Put in a medium-sized pot, add 2 inches of water, and bring to a boil. Simmer for 1 hour or until tender; you can use the beans whole or slightly mashed. Season with seasoning salt and set aside. Cook wild/brown rice and set aside. Lightly sauté the onion and garlic in macadamia oil. Add the greens and a small amount of water and steam-fry until just tender, about 5 minutes. Season with Bragg Liquid Aminos and set aside.

Lightly sauté the tofu in the same pan, adding seasoning salt to taste. Scoop out the tomatoes. Dice the scooped-out sections and set aside. Bake the hollowed-out tomatoes at 300 degrees for 5 to 10 minutes to warm. (Do not overbake or the tomatoes will get too soft.)

On individual serving plates, create a bottom "ring" of wild rice, with a second ring of seasoned black beans on top of it. Place a hollowed tomato in the center of the double-decker ring. Sprinkle tofu cubes around on top of the beans/rice at the base of the tomato and stuff the tomato with greens (spill the greens to overflow the top of the tomato if desired). Sprinkle the raw diced tomatoes on top of the greens, drizzle on a little Udo's Choice or olive oil, and serve.

Variation: If you like garlic, you can mix roasted garlic into the warm cooked brown rice before serving.

Robio's Burrito

SERVES 1

Donated by Robio.

This burrito would make a great meal anytime . . . even for breakfast. You can add or subtract and cut/slice/dice the items listed below to your own specifications. This recipe is very versatile, and you can add your own spin to it every time to make it delicious and entertaining.

1 sprouted-wheat, spelt, or grain tortilla
Organic refried beans
1 avocado
Herdez-brand salsa (hot, medium, or mild)
Lettuce
Tomato
Green pepper
Jalapeños
Onions
California white basmati rice, seasoned with Spanish spices
    (optional)

Place the refried beans directly down the middle of the tortilla, then add the other toppings as you like. Fold like a taco or roll up like a burrito.

✳ Energizer-Alkalizer Breakfast ✳

SERVES 2

Donated by Susan Lee Traft.

This breakfast keeps you going strong and feeling awesome for several hours.

¼ cup chopped red pepper
¼ cup chopped onion
1 clove minced garlic
About 2 cups mixed veggies (such as Swiss chard, broccoli, green
    beans, pea pods, zucchini, a few slices of carrot, etc.)
1–3 Tbs. golden flaxseeds, ground in a coffee grinder (tastes like
    bread crumbs)
1 Tbs. Udo's Choice Oil Blend
Bragg Liquid Aminos to taste

Bring water to a simmer under the steamer basket in pot. Add the red pepper, onion, garlic, and mixed veggies all at once into the steamer basket and cover. Lightly steam for no more than 5 minutes. Immediately remove the veggies from the heat and put into a salad bowl. Add the ground flaxseeds, oil, and Bragg. Mix well.

Coconut Curry Salmon Chowder

SERVES 4

This is a sweet, rich dish.

1 lb. fresh salmon
1 tsp. RealSalt
1–2 tsps. Garlic Herb Bread Seasoning (Spice Hunter)
1 yellow onion

8 stalks celery
6 carrots
2 cans coconut milk (I use Thai brand)
½ tsp. Thai green curry paste (I use Thai brand)
1–2 pkgs. powdered stevia (I use the kind with fiber; if you're using straight stevia, then use much less)
½ tsp. vanilla extract (no alcohol; I use Frontier brand)
1 cup fresh coconut
1 cup fresh peas from the pod (optional)
1 cup fresh spinach (optional)

Sprinkle the fish with some RealSalt and Garlic Herb Bread Seasoning, then steam-fry it or use some grape seed oil to fry it until cooked through but still moist. Cut into small bite-sized pieces and set aside. Cut the onion, celery, and carrots into bite-sized chunks, put them into a soup pot, and steam until bright and chewy. (Do not overcook.) Add the coconut milk, green curry paste, stevia, and vanilla, and stir to mix. Add the salmon. Take a third of the whole ingredients and puree in a blender, then return them to the soup for a thick colorful base. Add fresh coconut, fresh peas from the pod, and/or fresh spinach toward the end if you like, and warm before serving.

Steamed Fish and Greens

SERVES 4

1 lb. fresh salmon, trout, or red snapper fillet with skin on
RealSalt to taste
Garlic Herb Bread Seasoning (Spice Hunter)
1 Tbs. fresh ginger, cut into thin slices or grated
1 cup yellow chives
½ cup green chives
4 cups fresh kale
2 Tbs. Bragg Liquid Aminos

½–1 cup fresh coconut water (sweet) taken from a young fresh
coconut (I use a clean screwdriver and a hammer to make two
holes into the top of a coconut and pour the water out into a
measuring cup. Then I break open the coconut with the hammer
and use a sharp meat cleaver to get to the fresh coconut meat.)
½ cup cilantro

In a nonstick skillet, lay the fish, skin-side down, and steam-fry with
the lid on until it's cooked through but also moist. Halfway through,
take the lid off and sprinkle the fish with RealSalt and Garlic Herb
Bread Seasoning. When the fish is done, remove it to a plate and set
aside. Take the skin off the fish and discard, but leave any oils from
the fish in the pan. Place the thinly sliced ginger in the oiled pan and
cook until browned. Add all the other ingredients except the cilantro
and steam in the pan with the lid on until bright green and softened.
Add the fish and the cilantro back in and steam for 1 or 2 more minutes before serving.

Veggie Tofu Loaf (with Variations)

SERVES 6

*This is a wonderfully colorful and nutritious way to enjoy tofu at any
meal or even snack time. It's great steaming hot from the oven, or sliced
cold, or broken up over a salad. Use the firmest tofu type for best holding
results. I use Nigari–brand extra firm. For a binder, I use Mauk Family
Farms Wheat Free Crusts, a blend of gold and brown flaxseeds, sesame
seeds, and sunflower seeds, with garlic, onion, celery seeds, red bell pepper,
parsley, sea salt, and pepper, dehydrated at 105 degrees, and process them
in my food processor until they are a powder consistency. The flax, sunflower, and sesame seeds add extra flavor and healthy fats. This is also a
favorite dish served at the pH Miracle retreats.*

1 lb. firm or extra-firm tofu
½–1 tsp. RealSalt (or to taste)

5 tsps. Mexican Seasoning (Spice Hunter)
2 tsps. Vegetable Rub (Spice Hunter)
4 tsps. sun-dried tomatoes, minced (Melissa brand, packed in olive oil)
½ red bell pepper, diced
2 Tbs. diced celery
2 Tbs. diced soaked almonds
2 Tbs. Raw Wheat Free Crusts (Mauk Family Farms), ground to powder
Grape seed oil
Zip seasoning

Use a food processor to dice all the ingredients that need dicing. Then place all the ingredients in the food processor and pulse-chop until well mixed. Place on a grape-seed-oiled pan and mold into one larger loaf or two smaller loaves, about 2 inches in height. Brush some grape seed oil over the top of the loaf and sprinkle Zip over the top. Bake at 400 degrees for 20 to 30 minutes or until lightly browned on top. Serve warm or let it chill overnight, then slice and serve cold.

Variation 1: Garlic Veggie Tofu Loaf

1 lb. extra-firm Nigari tofu
½–1 tsp. RealSalt
2–4 roasted cloves garlic
2 Tbs. Spice House Dehydrated Veggie Granules
4 tsps. diced celery
4 tsps. diced red bell pepper
2 Tbs. ground Raw Wheat Free Crusts

Sprinkle Garlic Herb Bread Seasoning over the top.

Variation 2: Buckwheat Veggie Tofu Loaf

The binder for this variation is raw buckwheat flour. Grind raw buckwheat in your blender or grinder to make this flour fresh.

1 lb. extra-firm tofu
6 tsps. Vegetable Seasoning (Spice Hunter)
6 tsps. diced celery
3 tsps. red bell pepper
3 tsps. diced sun-dried tomato
5 tsps. Garlic Herb Bread Seasoning (Spice Hunter)
½–1 tsp. RealSalt
3 tsps. raw buckwheat, ground to flour

Top the loaf with 2 tsps. ground Raw Wheat Free Crusts.

Variation 3: Basil Veggie Tofu Loaf

1 lb. extra-firm Nigari tofu
½–1 tsp. RealSalt
4 tsps. diced celery
4 tsps. diced red bell pepper
2 Tbs. Vegetable Seasoning (Spice Hunter)
4 tsps. ground flaxseeds
4 tsps. ground soaked almonds
6–8 tsps. fresh-diced basil

Sprinkle Garlic Herb Bread Seasoning on top.

Variation 4: Quinoa Veggie Tofu Loaf

1 lb. extra-firm Nigari tofu
1 Tbs. Pesto Seasoning (Spice Hunter)
2 Tbs. diced celery
2 Tbs. diced red bell pepper
4 tsps. minced sun-dried tomato (packed in olive oil)
1 heaping Tbs. quinoa ground flour (grind in your blender)

Oil and place Spice House–brand dehydrated veggie granules on top.

Can't Get Enough Eggplant

SERVES 1–2

Donated by Myra Marvez.

1 eggplant
Finely chopped onion, size chosen according to taste and size of
    eggplant
Olive oil
Celtic Salt

Roast the eggplant on an open fire till it is mostly cooked. Cool and peel off all burned skin. Chop the eggplant into small pieces. Finely mince the onion. Place the eggplant in a bowl, add the onion, olive oil, salt, and mix well.

Cherry Tomatoes AvoRado Style

SERVES 2–4

This is a great appetizer or hors d'oeuvre, or it could be served as a salad course.

1 pt. cherry tomatoes
Juice of ½ lime
1 avocado
½ tsp. dried onion
1 Tbs. minced cilantro
⅛ tsp. Zip seasoning (Spice Hunter) (use more if you like it extra
    spicy)
⅛ tsp. RealSalt
Dehydrated vegetable granules (make your own or buy them)

Slice the tomato tops off and use a melon ball spoon to scoop out the seeds and pulp. Drain upside down on paper towels. In a food processor with an S blade, add the remaining ingredients and pulse-chop into a well-mixed, chunky consistency. Fill the tomato shells with the mixture and sprinkle dehydrated veggie granules on top. Serve chilled.

Doc Broc Stalks—Coyote Style

SERVES 4

The good news is that when Dr. Young first tried this dish, he thought he was eating fried potatoes! I love it when I can fake him out! The even better news is that this taste treat is actually made of broccoli. Even my fifteen-year-old Alex (our perpetual transitional boy) always asks for seconds and thirds of these.

6 long broccoli stalks, peeled and sliced thin (about ⅛ inch)
1 yellow onion, sliced thin and chopped
2 Tbs. grape seed oil
½–1 cup Creamy Tomato Soup (see page 193)
1–2 tsps. Garlic Herb Bread Seasoning (Spice Hunter)
1–2 tsps. Seafood Grill & Broil Seasoning (Spice Hunter)
1–2 tsps. Mesquite Seasoning (Spice Hunter)
½ tsp. ground yellow mustard
1–3 tsps. soy Parmesan dairy-free cheese (I use Soymage Vegan Parmesan)

Place the onion and broccoli stalk slices in a nonstick skillet and steam-fry for a few minutes until the veggies heat up and steam so they slip and slide around the pan. Add the grape seed oil and stir the veggies on high heat while they brown and become somewhat roasted. Once they are evenly fry-roasted, turn down the heat to low and add ½ cup of the Creamy Tomato Soup (more or less, depending on how much sauce you want in with your stalks; you can always add the other half later). Then sprinkle in seasonings to coat the stalks and onions. Stir well to distribute all the seasonings evenly. Last, sprinkle in soy Parmesan to taste and stir once more to mix well.

Doc Broc Brunch

SERVES 6

This is a hearty deep green dish that has plenty of crunch with the broccoli stalks and soaked almonds added. Perfect for a brunch or side dish.

3 large heads broccoli
1 lb. young green string beans
1 yellow onion
2 cloves fresh garlic
1 small bowl soaked almonds
Grape seed or olive oil
RealSalt to taste

Trim and peel the broccoli stalks, then cut the broccoli into bite-sized pieces. Trim and break the green beans into bite-sized pieces. Lightly steam the broccoli and green beans until bright green. In a food processor, pulse-chop the onion and garlic until fine; set aside. Put the soaked almonds into the food processor with an S blade and pulse-chop into almond slivers. In an electric skillet, place the oil, add the onion/garlic mixture, and sauté for a few minutes. Add the steamed broccoli/green beans and stir-fry to mix in with the onions and garlic. Add the slivered soaked almonds and continue to mix well. Put the lid on the skillet and continue to steam for a few minutes longer if softer veggies are desired. Add RealSalt to taste.

Doc Broc Casserole

SERVES 4–6

Florets from 2 large bunches broccoli (save the leaves and stalks, peeling and cleaning the stalks)
1 cup soft tofu
1 tsp. ground mustard seeds
1 small bunch fresh basil or tarragon, stemmed and minced
⅔ cup olive oil
1 pkg. Smart Ground by Lightlife (soy protein substitute)
1–2 cups roasted or soaked and re-dehydrated almonds for topping
RealSalt and Spice Hunter Zip to taste

Steam the broccoli florets with a little water in a covered pan for about 4 or 5 minutes, until the broccoli is bright green and just crisptender. In a food processor, process the broccoli leaves and stalks until very fine (scrape down the sides if necessary). Then add the soft tofu, mustard, and basil, and process. With the processor running, slowly add the olive oil until the mixture is well emulsified and creamy.

In a large electric skillet, heat a small amount of oil and add the Soy Smart Ground. Crumble it up and fry it for a couple of minutes, then add the steamed broccoli florets and pour the creamy sauce from the processor over the top; stir in well. Chop the almonds into small bits in the food processor for extra crunch, then sprinkle over the top of the broccoli mixture and serve. Or return the lid to the skillet and steam the mixture a bit to soften the almonds and broccoli more. Add RealSalt and Zip to taste.

Mary Jane's Super Simple Spaghetti

SERVES 2

Donated by Mary Jane Medlock.

1 medium spaghetti squash
2 medium ripe vine tomatoes, chopped
Juice of 1 small lemon
1–2 cloves fresh garlic, minced or chopped
2–3 Tbs. olive oil
Fresh-ground pepper
¼ tsp. oregano

Cut the spaghetti squash in half (clean out the seeds). In a baking dish, put the spaghetti squash face down and bake in a 375-degree oven for approximately 45 minutes or until done. Let cool for about 5 minutes. Using a fork, scoop out the spaghetti squash into a bowl. Add the remaining ingredients and toss. Eat warm or cold.

Veggies and Beans

SERVES 4–6

Donated by Linda Broadhead.

2 large beets, chopped
10 stalks asparagus, chopped
5–6 kale leaves, chopped
2 cups black beans (cooked)
1 tsp. cumin
¼ tsp. Jalapeno Chile Pepper (Spice Hunter)
1 tsp. Creole Seasoning (Spice Hunter)
2 Tbs. Bragg Liquid Aminos (or to taste)
2 cloves garlic, crushed

Juice of 1 lemon
1-inch chunk ginger, grated
2 scallions, chopped fine
1 raw yellow squash, cut into chunks

Steam the beets, asparagus, and kale until just tender. Mix the remaining ingredients and combine with the steamed veggies.

Salmon à la King or Queen

SERVES 4–6

Donated by Ray Sabo.

This is a good recipe for transitioning from yeasty starchy breads to yeast-free bread. The salmon and olive oil provide lots of healthy fats. The mixture of toppings and herbs make this recipe scrumptious.

½ cup olive oil
3–4 cloves garlic, minced
½–1 tsp. oregano (or to taste)
1–2 tsp. parsley (or to taste)
1–2 lbs. fresh salmon, cut into rectangular pieces
2–3 slices yeast-free bread, chopped very fine
Garlic powder
Soy butter
Parsley (to taste)
Thyme (to taste)

Preheat the oven to 300 to 350 degrees. Combine the olive oil, garlic, oregano, and parsley. Place the fish in a baking pan and brush with the herb mixture. Bake until it reaches your desired doneness; remove from the oven. Increase the temperature to broil. Mix the bread with the garlic powder and additional olive oil until it is a thick paste. Coat the top of the cooked salmon and broil just long enough to toast the topping. Make a sauce of melted soy butter seasoned with fresh parsley and thyme to taste, and drizzle over top of each piece just before serving. Garnish with a sprig of parsley.

Mama's Lasagna

SERVES 4–6

Individual plates of vegan lasagna with a variety of fresh veggies—you decide how much of each. Delicioso!

Almond cheese:
2 cups almonds, plumped
½ cup pine nuts
1 whole lemon
1½ tsps. RealSalt
2 tsps. dried basil (or several leaves fresh basil)
3 garlic cloves

Red sauce:
1½ cups dried tomatoes
4 cups water
1 Tbs. oregano
1 Tbs. basil
1 Tbs. thyme
1 Tbs. rosemary (or Italian seasonings of your choice)
2 tsps. RealSalt (or to taste)
Up to 10 cloves garlic (to your liking), raw or roasted

Putting it all together:
Spinach
Cucumber, thinly sliced
Eggplant, thinly sliced (optional)
Tomato, thinly sliced
Unsweetened dried coconuts, pulverized in a Vita-Mix

To make the almond cheese, place the almonds in a blender or Vita-Mix with just enough water to almost cover them. Add remaining ingredients and blend until creamy. Set aside for a while to let the flavors mingle.

To make the red sauce, blend all the ingredients in a blender or Vita-Mix and let stand to allow the flavors to mingle. Warm just before using.

To assemble the lasagna, layer a plate with a bed of spinach to define the serving size. Cover with a layer of cucumber, then eggplant (if using), and tomato. Pour almond cheese on top, and cover with another layer of spinach. Then pour red sauce over it all, enough to cover the sides as well. Dust the top with the "cocoparm cheese."

Fourth of July in a Bun

SERVES 4

Donated by Myra Marvez.

This is a wonderful "hot dog," using sprouted-wheat tortillas for a bun.

1 cup walnuts
1 cup plumped almonds
1 cup sunflower seeds
⅓ cup dried onion flakes
1½ tsps. RealSalt (or to taste)
2 stalks celery, with leafy greens on top
Juice of 1 lemon
1 head lettuce, chopped
2–3 tomatoes, chopped
4 sprouted-wheat tortillas

Place the nuts, seeds, onion flakes, salt, celery, and lemon juice in a food processor and grind until well blended. Form the mixture into 6-inch-long cylinder-shaped "hot dogs" and put in a food dehydrator overnight on low heat. To serve, warm the hot dogs and place them in folded tortillas, filling with lettuce, tomatoes, and dressing of your choice.

Happy-Chick Burgers

SERVES 2–4

Donated by Myra Marvez.

Because the chick is still alive, and so happy . . .

1 carton soft silken tofu
⅓ cup olive oil
3 green scallions
1 cup shredded carrots
1 cup shredded celery
1 tsp. baking powder
½ cup flour
1 tsp. RealSalt

Mix all the ingredients in a food processor, then form into patties. Cook in a low oven for half an hour, or fry in grape seed oil over low heat, until golden brown.

Spicy Nutty Nuggets

SERVES 4–6

Donated by Myra Marvez.

Serve in sprouted-wheat tortillas, cut up and mix into salad, or just pop them into your mouth for a snack!

1 cup plumped almonds
1 cup pecans
1 cup sunflower seeds
1 medium onion
2 garlic cloves
1 jalapeño
1 cup fresh parsley
1½ tsps. RealSalt
½ cup dried tomatoes
¾ cup ground dark flaxseeds

Put all the ingredients except the ground flaxseeds into a food processor and process until well blended and pasty. Form into nugget shapes, then roll in the ground flaxseeds. Place on dehydrator trays and dry overnight on low heat.

True Golden Nuggets

SERVES 2–4

Donated by Myra Marvez.

Serve with Garlic French Dressing (see page 242) and a side of jicama fries.

2 cups plumped almonds
1 cup water (more or less)

1 medium onion
1 lemon
1 tsp. fresh basil
1 tsp. fresh oregano
1 tsp. fresh thyme
1 tsp. RealSalt
½–1 cup ground golden flaxseed powder

Put the plumped almonds into a blender with just enough water to almost cover them. Blend until the consistency is pasty and still moist—add water if needed. Add the onion, whole lemon, basil, oregano, thyme, and salt and blend again. Form into little nugget-shaped patties. Put the ground flaxseed powder into plastic bag. Put the nuggets inside and shake until well coated. Place on dehydrator sheets and dehydrate overnight on low heat.

Colorful Cabbage

SERVES 4

Cabbage is considered one of the most powerful therapeutic foods in the world. Many studies have linked eating cabbage with a reduction of cancer, especially colon cancer. Also, cabbage juice has been proven to help heal stomach ulcers and prevent stomach cancer.

2 cups red cabbage, thinly sliced
2 cups green cabbage, thinly sliced
1 carrot, grated
1 red pepper, slivered
1 yellow pepper, slivered
1 green pepper, slivered
1 orange pepper, slivered
4 Tbs. chopped scallions
4 Tbs. minced parsley
¼ cup lemon juice

3 Tbs. water
1 Tbs. oil (extra-virgin olive, flaxseed, or Udo's Choice)
1–2 tsps. dried red chili pepper
Dash of Bragg Liquid Aminos

In a bowl, combine all the ingredients. Toss thoroughly and let the flavors mix for at least half an hour before serving.

SNACKS/DESSERTS

These recipes are healthy ways to enjoy a dessert or snack that won't contribute to high acidity. They will also help when blood sugar levels drop too low.

Onion-Flax Crackers

SERVES 6–8

Donated by Roxy Boelz. Third place, pH Miracle Recipe Contest.

2 cups sprouted sunflower seeds
1 cup chopped onion
½ cup fresh lemon juice or grapefruit juice (not sweet)
1 garlic clove
¼ cup golden flaxseeds
2 Tbs. raw almond butter or tahini
RealSalt to taste
¼ cup fennel seeds, sesame seeds, or caraway seeds
½ cup filtered water

Puree all the ingredients in a food processor. Pour onto Teflex sheets for the dehydrator. Dehydrate at 105 to 110 degrees for 12 hours or to the desired crispness. Periodically score the batter as it dehydrates so you can separate more easily into crackers when done.

Halvah Coconut Freezer Balls

SERVES 12

Donated by Debra Jenkins.
First place, pH Miracle Recipe Contest,
Transitional Recipes Category.

1 Tbs. Garden of Life coconut oil
3 Tbs. raw tahini
1 Tbs. vanilla extract
3 Tbs. fresh-grated coconut
⅛ tsp. stevia
2 Tbs. spelt flour

Melt the coconut oil and mix all the ingredients together. Drop teaspoonfuls onto a small cookie sheet or plate. Freeze for 15 to 20 minutes. Transfer to a freezer bag or container and eat as a luscious, quick dessert right from the freezer or fridge.

Variation: Use 3 Tbs. almond butter in place of tahini.

Coconut Macadamia Nut Cookies

SERVES 8

Donated by Debra Jenkins.
First place, pH Miracle Recipe Contest,
Transitional Recipes Category.

½ cup fresh-ground spelt flour (from spelt flakes; I use my old coffee grinder)
½ cup fresh-grated coconut
¼ cup chopped macadamia nuts
½ tsp RealSalt
¼ tsp. nutmeg
½ tsp. cardamom
1 tsp. cinnamon
Stevia to taste (I use 2–3 pkgs. or ¼ tsp. stevia powder)
4 Tbs. Garden of Life coconut oil
Egg substitute equivalent to 2 eggs (see below—make a double recipe)
1½ Tbs. nonalcoholic Frontier vanilla extract

Mix the dry ingredients together. Melt the coconut oil and mix with the egg substitute and vanilla. Pour the liquid ingredients over the dry ingredients and mix well. Drop onto cookie sheets and press very flat. Bake at 350 degrees for 15 to 20 minutes. Cool completely.

Egg Substitutes

Egg Substitute 1

EQUIVALENT TO ABOUT 1 EGG

⅓ cup water
1 Tbs. flaxseeds

Gently boil the water and flaxseeds in a saucepan for about 5 minutes. Look for the consistency of a raw egg white. Do *not* use high heat or the mixture will gel. You might want to strain this before using, depending on the recipe you are using. It is not necessary for Coconut Macadamia Nut Cookies.

Egg Substitute 2

EQUIVALENT TO ABOUT 1 EGG

⅔ cup water
1–2 Tbs. agar flakes

Stir to combine.

Egg Substitute 3

EQUIVALENT TO ABOUT 1 EGG

Use arrowroot flour in place of the agar or flaxseeds in either recipe above. (There's no need to boil it.)

Pumpkin Crème Pie

SERVES 6–8

Donated by Debra Jenkins.
First place, pH Miracle Recipe Contest,
Transitional Recipes Category.

1 pkg. (12 oz.) silken tofu
2 cups fresh-pureed pumpkin (or yams)
2 tsp. Frontier alcohol-free vanilla extract
2 tsps. cinnamon
¼ tsp. RealSalt
¾ tsp. nutmeg
¼ tsp. cloves
½ tsp. ginger
¼ tsp. white stevia powder or 2–3 pkgs. stevia powder
**3 Tbs. psyllium (agar powder or flakes can be substituted for psyl-
  lium, as well)**
1 recipe Almond Nut Piecrust (see below)

Mix the tofu, pumpkin, vanilla, cinnamon, salt, nutmeg, cloves, ginger, and stevia powder together in a food processor till smooth and
creamy. (Add more spices or stevia if you like, or use fewer spices for
a milder pie.) Last, add the psyllium and blend. Scoop into the prepared crust and chill for at least an hour. Top with Nutty Crème
Topping (see page 231) or Tofu "Whipped Cream" (see page 230).

Almond Nut Piecrust

MAKES ONE 9-INCH CRUST

Donated by Debra Jenkins.
First place, pH Miracle Recipe Contest,
Transitional Recipes Category.

½ cup fresh spelt flakes, ground into flour (I use my old coffee
    grinder)
½ cup ground almonds
¼ cup fresh-ground flax meal
1 Tbs. arrowroot powder
½ tsp. ground cinnamon
⅛ tsp. ground cloves
1 pkg. stevia powder
1 tsp. Frontier alcohol-free vanilla extract
2 Tbs. Garden of Life coconut oil (melted)
2 Tbs. water

Combine the dry ingredients in a mixing bowl. Combine the vanilla,
oil, and water and pour over the dry ingredients. Mix well. Transfer
the mixture to a 9-inch pie plate. Press the mixture firmly into place
with your fingers, making sure to cover the bottom and sides of the
plate. For an unfilled piecrust, bake the empty shell at 350 degrees
for 18 to 20 minutes or until lightly brown. Cool and fill with pie
filling. For a filled piecrust, first bake the empty crust for 10 minutes,
then fill and finish baking the pie per recipe.

Variation: Replace the flax meal with ground coconut.

Avocado Coconut Key Lime Pie

SERVES 6–8

Donated by Debra Jenkins.
First place, pH Miracle Recipe Contest,
Transitional Recipes Category.

8 oz. silken tofu
½ cup fresh lime juice
1 tsp. Frontier nonalcoholic vanilla extract
2 Tbs. fresh-grated coconut
⅛ tsp. RealSalt
1 small or ½ medium avocado
⅛ tsp. powdered white stevia
⅛ tsp. grated lime peel
3 Tbs. psyllium flakes or agar flakes
1 recipe Almond Nut Piecrust (see above)

Add all the ingredients (except the psyllium flakes and lime peel) to a food processor or blender and mix till smooth and creamy. Add more stevia to taste, if desired. Fold in the psyllium flakes and lime peel. Spoon into the already prepared Almond Nut Piecrust. Sprinkle coconut and chopped walnuts or pecans over the top as a garnish and chill in the refrigerator for 1 to 2 hours.

Variation: Add 6 Tbs. coconut milk to the first batch of ingredients, and reduce the psyllium to 1 Tbs.

AB&J Sandwiches with Red Pepper Jelly

SERVES 1–2

Donated by Cheri Freeman.
Third place, pH Miracle Recipe Contest.

Sprouted-wheat tortillas
Almond butter
Red Pepper Jelly (see below)

Warm the tortillas and cut into quarters. Spread on almond butter and Red Pepper Jelly. Makes little triangle-sandwiches, a great
snack!

Red Pepper Jelly

SERVES 4 (MAKES 1½ CUPS)

This keeps for a few days in the fridge, or you can freeze it to use later.

2 red bell peppers
½ cup plus 3 Tbs. water
30 drops stevia (or to taste)
4 tsps. Pomona's Universal Pectin
4 tsps. calcium water (packet comes with pectin)

Grind or puree the peppers in a blender or food processor with
3 Tbs. of the water. Add stevia to taste. Pour into a bowl. Prepare the
calcium water, and stir into the pepper mixture. Bring ½ cup of
water just to a boil and pour into a food processor or blender.
Quickly add the pectin and blend. (You must work fast, or the pectin
will form globs.) Quickly pour the pectin mixture into the bowl with
the pepper mixture and stir well. Pour into glass jar and refrigerate.
It will gel completely in a couple of hours.

Red Pepper Dessert Boats

SERVES 4–6

Donated by Eric Prouty.
Second place, pH Miracle Recipe Contest,
Alkalizing Recipes Category.

1½ cups soaked sunflower seeds
1 Tbs. pumpkin seed oil
1 tsp. cinnamon
7 drops liquid stevia mixed with 1 tsp. water
2 red bell peppers

Use a Green Star/Green Life or Champion juicer with a plug attachment for nut butters to process the sunflower seeds. Mix in the oil, cinnamon, and stevia/water. Slice the red bell peppers in half vertically, core, and cut in slices top to bottom, ½ to 1 inch wide. Spread the slices with the sunflower seed mixture.

Holiday Almonds

SERVES 2–4

Donated by JoAnn Efeney.

1 cup water
½ cup almonds
⅛ tsp. ground cloves
⅛ tsp. ground ginger
⅛ tsp. ground nutmeg
⅛ tsp. ground cinnamon

Put the almonds into the water and add the spices. Let the mixture set overnight, then stir and enjoy.

Variation: After the almonds soak in the spices, drain and dehydrate. You'll get a nice extra-crunchy snack with a hint of spiciness.

Deliciously Dill Petaled Cucumbers

SERVES 4–6

2 English cucumbers
Juice of 1 large lime
1 tsp. Deliciously Dill seasoning (Spice Hunter)
Small amount of water, if needed
RealSalt to taste

Run fork prongs along the cucumbers to create a petaled look, then slice ¼ inch thick. Place the sliced cucumber in shallow bowl with the juice, dill seasoning, and RealSalt. Marinate in the fridge for at least half an hour. Serve chilled.

Veggie Crispy Crackers with Soy Sprouts Powder

SERVES 4–6

These are great for a crunchy cracker snack, or broken up and sprinkled over a salad like croutons.

3 carrots
1 small carton cherry or grape tomatoes
3 sun-dried tomatoes packed in olive oil
1 tsp. piece fresh ginger
3 stalks celery
2 tomatillos
⅓ yam, peeled

1 yellow crookneck squash
⅓ cup fresh mixed herbs, such as rosemary, oregano, tarragon,
   thyme, cilantro, parsley, and basil
½ cup sprouted buckwheat (I use a 2-day sprout: Soak raw buckwheat for at least 6 hours, and rinse for 2 days)
⅓ cup flaxseeds (you don't have to soak them)
1–2 heaping Tbs. soy sprouts powder

Put the first nine ingredients into your food processor and pulse-
chop until all the veggies are mixed well, moist, and diced. Alterna-
tively, you can place all nine ingredients through a Green Power
juicer with the blank attachment and put the moist pulp into a mixing bowl. Add the sprouted buckwheat, flaxseeds, and soy powder
and mix well. Pour the mixture out onto plastic-sheet-lined trays for
the dehydrator and pat or spatula the mixture out into a large square
or rectangle. Dehydrate for 4 to 5 hours at 90 to 95 degrees, and then
cut into smaller squares (3 by 3 inches) and transfer to mesh-lined
trays for continued drying until crisp (about 4 hours more). Or let
the crackers continue drying through the night and break the finished pieces up into small pieces in the morning. If done right, these
can last up to a month in an airtight container, though I'm sure they
will be eaten up long before that!

Bird Nest Crackers

Serves 4–6

*These are fun to place on the top of a bowl of soup right before you serve it.
I form these crackers into little nest shapes and put some fresh peas from
the pod in them for hors d'oeuvres. Plain, these crackers travel well. Being
dehydrated, they offer concentrated nutrition.*

2 yellow crookneck squash
2 zucchinis

½ tsp. RealSalt
½ tsp. All Purpose Chef's Shake (Spice Hunter) or seasoning of
   choice
2 tsp. Vegetable Seasoning (Spice Hunter) or seasoning of choice

Clean the squash and zucchinis, taking care to cut any scars off the skin. Shred in a food processor and combine with the spices. Spoon out onto Teflon sheets. You can make them lacier by loosely placing the mixture on the sheet in a small circle, which will dry like a lacy cracker with holes showing, or you can pack the mixture tightly and form little nests to create a denser cracker nest. Dehydrate overnight to 24 hours and store in an airtight container.

Variation: Experiment with added veggies, seeds, or nuts, such as soaked almonds, sunflower seeds, sweet peas, shredded carrots, jalapeños, and flaxseeds. You can also use your own favorite seasonings to get the flavors you like best.

Edamame Beans

SERVES 2–4

Put the whole pod into your mouth, bite down, and slide out the beans for a yummy snack or side dish.

1 12- or 16-oz. pkg. frozen edamame (soybeans)
Oil
RealSalt
Seasoning of your choice

Boil the edamame as per the directions on the package. Strain, then dash a few squirts of olive oil or other healthy oil, some RealSalt, or your favorite Spice Hunter seasonings over the edamame pods. We like Vegetable Rub or Garlic Herb Bread Seasoning. Good served warm or cold.

Sprouted Buckwheat Flatties

SERVES 6

These are thin and crustlike in texture. They are marvelous as a raw (low-heat-dehydrated) pizza crust. You can dry them big in large rounds or break them up and use them as crackers or sandwich pieces. Experiment with this basic recipe and come up with versions of your own! You will need a good dehydrator and a food processor, as well as sprouting equipment. The preparation for these flatties may seem like a lot of time and work, but once you get the hang of it, it will surely be worth it. I triple and quadruple this recipe to fill my entire Excalibur (nine trays) with flatties. These flatties will stay fresh in a Ziploc bag or Tupperware container for as long as a month. Great for hiking and camping trips, biking, or on a long flight. Our grandson CharLee is cutting his first teeth on these alkaline crackers!

1⅓ cups carrot pulp or shredded carrot; or raw yam, squash, or zucchini; or a mixture of those
⅓ cup Essential Balance oil (Omega Nutrition or Arrowhead Mills)
2 tsp. RealSalt
2 tsp. Garlic Herb Bread Seasonings (Spice Hunter)
1 tsp. All Purpose Chef's Shake (Spice Hunter)
3 cups sprouted buckwheat (I use a 2-day sprout: soak raw buckwheat for 6–8 hours, and rinse for 2 days)
2–3 sun-dried tomatoes (optional)
⅓–⅔ cup flaxseeds (you don't have to soak)
¼–⅓ cup water (optional)

Pulse-chop the veggie pulp, oil, salt, and seasonings in a food processor to mix well. Then add the remaining ingredients and continue to process until you get a thick batter that is quite smooth. (You could also stop mixing earlier if you prefer a coarse batter with more whole buckwheat sprouts.) While the food processor is running, you can add the water if you feel the batter needs to be thinned some to make spreading easier.

Pour or scoop the mixture out onto plastic-lined trays for dehydration. Use a spatula to help spread out the batter so your flattie is ¼ to ½ inch thick. Then dehydrate at 90 to 100 degrees overnight or for 7 to 8 hours. Carefully lift the flatties, transferring them to a mesh-lined tray, and continue dehydrating until totally crisp and dry, about 4 to 6 more hours.

Variation: Experiment with other seasonings in place of the Chef's Shake, like 1 Tbs. soy sprouts powder, 1 tsp. green powder, Italian pizza seasoning, 2 Tbs. fresh basil, or whatever you like best.

Super Soy Pudding

SERVES 2

This is a great way to have a delicious snack while staying alkaline. We even eat this wonderful pudding for breakfast or in place of one of the soups on the liquid feast. It is high in good fats, vitamin E, calcium, and potassium (from the almond milk and avocado), as well as high in good proteins (from the Super Soy Powder).

1 cup Fresh Silky Almond Milk (see page 183) or coconut milk
1 avocado
1 whole lime, peeled
2 scoops sprouted soy powder
1 pkg. stevia
6–8 ice cubes

Put all the ingredients in a blender and blend on high until rich and smooth and puddinglike.

Variations: For Coconut Super Soy Pudding, use the coconut milk, and add 2 Tbs. of unsweetened dried coconut granules to the mix. Sprinkle some coconut over the top before serving.

For Lemon Super Soy Pudding, use a lemon instead of a lime.

For Grapefruit Super Soy Pudding, use the juice from ½ grapefruit instead of a lime.

For Super Green Super Soy Pudding, add ½ scoop of green powder or 1 cup fresh baby spinach.

For Ginger Super Soy Pudding, add a pinch or two of fresh-grated ginger.

For Cinnamon Super Soy Pudding, add a pinch or two of cinnamon and nutmeg to the mix, and sprinkle more on top.

For Nutty Super Soy Pudding, add chopped raw almonds (or pecans or macadamias, or whatever you like).

For Super Soy Pops, pour your favorite variation into pop molds and freeze. Or use small paper cups or ice cube trays, adding pop sticks or toothpicks when the mixture is partially frozen.

For Super Soy Slushy, freeze your favorite variation in ice cube trays, thaw slightly, and chop up.

Pumpkin Slush-elicious

SERVES 2–4

Donated by Linda Broadhead.

1 cup coconut milk
1 cup pumpkin puree
1 tsp. Spice Hunter Pumpkin Pie Spice
2 tsps. stevia (Stevita brand; use spoonable type)

⅛ tsp. RealSalt
Ice cubes to reach 5 cups in blender

Place all the ingredients in a blender or Vita-Mix and blend until smooth.

Almond Slush-elicious

SERVES 1–2

Donated by Linda Broadhead.

½ cup coconut milk
4 ice cubes
1 Tbs. raw almond butter
20 drops stevia (Stevita brand)
¼ tsp. Frontier Anise Flavor (no alcohol)

Place all the ingredients in a blender or Vita-Mix and blend until slushy.

Resources

The pH Miracle Healing Centers, Innerlight, and the Youngs

For referrals for live blood analysis and the Mycotoxic/Oxidative Stress Test (MOST), or health retreats or consultations, contact The pH Miracle Center at 760-751-8321. This is also the place to call for information about products used in this book that this resources section does not provide:

The pH Miracle Healing Centers

16390 Dia Del Sol
Valley Center, CA 92082
760-751-8321
Fax: 760-751-8324

www.thephmiraclecenter.com

For general information, recipes, articles and testimonials: www.thephmiracle.us.

For further video education on the New Biology and the pH Miracle lifestyle and diet: www.innerlightmotion.com.

Supplements

- InnerLight, Inc., 867 East 2260 South, Provo, UT 84606. You can order the nutritional supplements described in *The pH Miracle for Diabetics* at www.innerlightinc.com.
- Source Natural, Inc., 19 Janis Way, Scotts Valley, CA 95066; 800-815-2333; www.sourcenaturals.com.
- Solaray: Nutraceutical Corporation, 1400 Kearns Boulevard, Second Floor, Park City, UT 84060; 800-669-8877; www. nutraceutical.com.

- Green Kamut Corporation, 1965 Freeman, Long Beach, CA 90804.

Food

- California avocados, organically grown on our ranch, picked fresh off the tree and shipped to you next day: 760-751-8321; www.ranchavorado.com or www.thephmiraclecenter.com.
- Extra-virgin coconut oil: Garden of Life, 800-622-8986; www.gardenoflifeusa.com.
- New Frontier flavorings bottled in oil (without alcohol): www.frontiercoop.com.
- Pomona's Universal Pectin is available at health food or grocery stores, Whole Foods, or from Workstead Industries, P.O. Box 1083, Greenfield, MA 01302; 413-772-6816.
- Heat Wave Seasoning from the Cape Herb and Spice Company, distributed by Profile Products: P.O. Box 140, Maple Valley, WA 98038; 425-432-4300; www.elements-of-spice.com.
- Litehouse Spice Company: www.litehousefoods.com.
- Spice House dehydrated tomato powder and veggie granules: www.thespicehouse.com.
- Mauk Family Farms Raw Wheat Free Crusts: www.maukfamilyfarms.com.
- RealSalt: Redmond Minerals, Inc., 800-367-7258; www.realsalt.com.
- For a wonderful, easy-to-get-started program on sprouting, kits in different sizes, instructions on how to sprout, information on nutritional aspects of different seeds, single seeds, and seed mixes: Life Sprouts, P.O. Box 150, Hiram, UT 94321; 435-245-3891.
- There are many organic food distributors, many of which are based in California with its year-round growing climate. Here's one I like: Diamond Organics, P.O. Box 2159, Freedom, CA 95019; 888-674-2642; fax orders: 888-888-6777; e-mail: organics@diamondorganics.com.

- Pacific Foods of Oregon, Tualatin, OR 97062; 503-692-9666; www.pacificfoods.com.
- Udo's Choice: Flora, Inc., Lyden, WA 98264; 800-446-2110; www.udoerasmus.com or www.florainc.com.
- Essential Balance/Omega Nutrition Oil: Arrowhead Mills, Vancouver, BC V5L 1P5; 800-661-3529; www.omeganutrition. com.
- Image Foods, Inc., 350 Cambridge Avenue, Suite 350, Palto Alto, CA 94306; www.imagefoods.com.
- For workshops on preparing alkalizing meals: Shelley Young's Academy of Culinary Arts, The pH Miracle Healing Center, Dia Del Sol, Valley Center, CA 92082; 760-751-8321; www. thephmiraclecenter.com.
- Recommended brands: Sweet Leaf stevia with fiber; Pacific free-range organic chicken broth and yeast-free vegetable broth; Pomi strained tomatoes with no preservatives, additives, or vinegar. White Wave baked seasoned tofu; Veat gourmet baked seasoned tofu; Gardenburgers; Boca Burgers; Spice Hunter spice combinations.

Equipment

- pH strips: http://thephmiracle.us/products.html.
- Cellerciser mini-tramp: The pH Miracle Healing Center; for more information, 760-751-8321.
- Infrared sauna: Nova, http://www.novacompanies.com/ Merchant2/merchant.mvc?Screen=CTGY&CategoryCode= THERASAUNA.
- LiquidLight Electro-Magnetic MicroIonization Water Machine (a product we developed): Visit www.thephmiracle.us for more information.
- One place you can buy a glucose monitoring system is Health-Max at 206-362-1111 or www.healthmax.net.
- Vita-Mix blender with the plunger: Vita-Mix, 8615 Usher Road, Cleveland, OH 44138-2199; 800-848-2649.
- Green Power, Green Star, Green Life juices: orders 888-254-7336; inquiries 562-940-4240; www.greenpower.com.

Cutting Edge

The Cutting Edge Catalogue carries many items in the category of health technology, including pH meters, water systems, and books:

Cutting Edge Catalogue
P.O. Box 5034
Southampton, NY 11969
Orders: 800-497-9516
Information: 516-287-3813
Fax: 516-287-3112

www.cutcat.com

E-mail: cutcat@i-2000.com

Books

- *Dr. Bernstein's Diabetes Solution* by Richard K. Bernstein, M.D., F.A.C.N., F.A.C.E., C.W.S.
- *Reversing Diabetes* by Julian Whitaker, M.D.
- *Victory Over Diabetes* by William H. Philpott, M.D., and Dwight K. Kalita, Ph.D.
- *The Diabetes Cure* by Vern Cherewatenko, M.D.
- *Diabetes: The Facts That Let You Regain Control of Your Life* by Charles Kilo, M.D., and Joseph R. Williamson, M.D.
- *The First Year Type 2 Diabetes: An Essential Guide for the Newly Diagnosed* by Gretchen Becker
- *The Diabetes Sourcebook* by Diana W. Guthrie, R.N., Ph.D., and Richard A. Guthrie, M.D.
- *Combat Syndrome X, Y and Z . . .* by Stephen Holt, M.D.
- *Natural Treatments for Diabetes* (*The Natural Pharmacist* series) by Kathi Head, N.D.
- *The Blood and Its Third Anatomical Element* by Antoine Bechamp
- *Soy Smart Health* by Neil Solomon, M.D., Ph.D.
- *Understanding Acid-Base* by Benjamin Abelow, M.D.
- *Fats That Heal and Fats That Kill* by Udo Erasmus

- *Slow Burn: Slow Down, Burn Fat, and Unlock the Energy Within* by Stu Mittleman
- *Muscles in Minutes* by Mike Mentzer
- *Static Contraction Training* by Peter Sisco and John R. Little
- *The Complete Book of Massage* by Claire Maxwell-Hudson
- *The Touch That Heals* by William N. Brown, Ph.D., N.D., D.Sc.
- *The Clay Cure* by Ran Knishinsky
- *Herbal Nutritional Medications* by Robert O. Young, Ph.D.

References

Airola, P. *How to Get Well.* Phoenix: Health Plus Publications, 1974, p. 260.

Albert, M. Vitamin B_{12} synthesis by human small intestinal bacteria. *Nature,* 1980; 283: 781.

Albrink, J.J., Davidson, P. C., and Newman, T. Lipid lowering effect of a very high-carbohydrate high-fiber diet. *Diabetes,* 1980; 26(suppl. 1): 324.

———. 1977. Effect of carbohydrate restriction and high-carbohydrate diets on men with chemical diabetes. *American Journal of Clinical Nutrition,* 1977; 30: 402–8.

American Diabetes Association. Diabetes facts and figures; http://www.diabetes.org/ada/facts/asp.

Anderson, J. *Plant Fiber in Foods.* Lexington: HCF Diabetes Research Foundation, 1981.

———. Independence of the effects of cholesterol and degree of saturation of the fat in the diet of serum cholesterol in man. *American Journal of Clinical Nutrition,* 1976; 29: 1184.

Anderson, R.A. Elevated intakes of supplemental chromium improve glucose and insulin variables in individuals with Type II diabetes. *Diabetes,* 1997; 46(11): 1786–91.

———. Effects of lifestyle activity vs. structured aerobic exercise in obese women. A randomized trial. *Journal of the American Medical Association,* Jan. 27, 1999; 281(4): 335–40.

———. Chromium as an essential nutrient for humans. *Regulatory Toxicology and Pharmacology,* 1997; 26(pts. 1, 2): S35–S41.

———. Chromium metabolism and its role in disease processes in man. *Clinical Physiology Biochemistry,* 1986; 4: 31–41.

Ayer, E., and Gauld, W. A. G. *Science,* April 12, 1946.

Aykroyd, W., and Doughty, J. *Wheat in the Human Nutrition.* Rome: FAO of the U.N., 1970; 19.

Bailey, H. *Vitamin E: Your Key to a Healthy Heart.* New York: Arc Books, 1971, pp. 97–98.

Baker, S. Evidence regarding the minimal daily requirement of dietary vitamin B_{12}. *American Journal of Clinical Nutrition,* 1981; 34: 2423.

Baldwa, V. S., et al. Clinical trial in patients with diabetes mellitus of an insulin-like compound obtained from plant sources. *Uppsala Journal of Medical Sciences,* 1977; 82: 39–41.

Bamard, J. Responses of non-insulin-dependent diabetic patients to an intensive program of diet and exercise. *Diabetes Care,* 1982; 5: 370.

Bamdt, R. Regression and progression of early femerol atherosclerosis in treated hyperlipoproteinemic patients. *Annals of International Medicine,* 1977; 86: 139.

Bantle, J. Postprandial glucose and insulin responses to meals containing different carbohydrate in normal and diabetic subjects. *New England Journal of Medicine,* 1983; 309: 7.

Barton, B.S. *Collection for an Essay Towards a Materia Medica of the United States,* 3rd ed., with additions. Philadelphia, printed for Edward Earle and Co., 1810.

Baskaran, K., et al. Antidiabetic effect of a leaf extract from Gymnema sylvestre in non-insulin-dependent diabetes mellitus patients. *Journal of Ethnopharmacology,* 1990; 30: 295–305.

Basta, L., Williams, C., Kioschos, J., Michael, S., and Arthur, A. Regression of atherosclerotic stenosing lesions of the renal arteries and spontaneous cure of systemic hypertension through control of hyperlidemia. *American Journal of Medicine,* 1976; 61: 420–23.

Basu, T. K., et al. Serum Vitamin A and retinol-binding protein in patients with insulin-dependent diabetes mellitus. *American Journal of Clinical Nutrition,* 1989; 50: 329–31.

Beaudeaux, J. L., et al. Enhanced susceptibility of low-density lipoprotein to in vitro oxidation in Type I and Type II diabetic patients. *Clinica Chimica Acta,* 1995; 239: 131–41.

Bennion, L. J., and Grundy, S. M. Effects of diabetes mellitus on cholesterol metabolism in man. *New England Journal of Medicine,* 1977; 296: 1365–71.

Bersin, T., Mueller, A., and Schwarz, H. Substances contained in crataegus oxyacantha. III. A Heptahydroxyflaven glycoside. *Arzeimettek-Forschungen,* 1955, pp. 490–91.

Berson, S. Plasma insulin in health and disease. *American Journal of Medicine,* 1961; 31: 874.

Biard, J. F., Verbist, J. F., Boterff, J., Rages, G., and Lecocq, M. M. Seaweeds of French Atlantic coast with antibacterial and antifungal compounds. *Planta Medica* (suppl.), 1980; 136–51.

Bierenbaum, M. L., Fleishman, A. I., Dunn, J., and Arnold, J. Possible acidic water factor in coronary heart disease. *Lancet,* 1975; 1: 1008–10.

Bingley, P. J., et al. Combined analysis of autoantibodies improves perdition of IDDM in islet cell antibody-positive relatives. *Diabetes,* 1994; 43: 1304–10.

Bland, J. *The Accessory Nutrients,* vols. 1 and 2. New Canaan, CT: Keats Publishing, Inc., 1982.

Borden, G., et al. Effects of vanadyl sulfate on carbohydrate and lipid metabolism in patients with non-insulin-dependent diabetes mellitus. *Metabolism,* 1996; 45(9): 1130–35.

Boyer, J. Exercise therapy in hypertensive men. *Journal of the American Medical Association,* 1970; 211: 1668.

Brunzell, J. Improved glucose tolerance with high carbohydrate feeding in mild diabetes. *New England Journal of Medicine,* 1971; 284: 521.

Burkitt, D. Dietary fiber and diseases. *Journal of the American Medical Association,* 1974; 229: 1068.

———. Some diseases characteristic of modern Western civilization. *British Medical Journal,* 1973; 1: 274.

———. Varicose veins, deep vein thrombosis, and hemorrhoids: Epidemiology and suggested aetiology. *British Medical Journal,* 1972; 2: 556.

Burkitt, D. P., and Trowell, H. C. *Refined Carbohydrate Foods and Disease: Some Implications of Dietary Fibre.* New York: Academic Press, 1975.

Cameron, N.E., et al. Effects of alpha-lipoic acid on neurovascular function in diabetic rats. *Diabetologia*, 1998; 41: 390–99.

Campbell, P., et al. Pathogenesis of the dawn phenomenon in patients with insulin-dependent diabetes mellitus. *New England Journal of Medicine*, 1985; 312: 1473–79.

Canfield, W. K., and Doisy, R. J., eds. Evidence of an unrecognized metabolic defect in diabetic subjects. *Diabetes*, 1975; 24(2): 406 (abstract).

Canham, R. S. Excretion of sodium, potassium, magnesium, and iron in human sweat and the relation of each to balance and requirements. *Journal of Nutrition*, 1962; 19: 407–15.

Carlson, Wade. *The Rejuvenated Vitamin*. New York, Award Books, 1970, p. 21.

Carmel, R. Nutritional vitamin B_{12} deficiency, possible contributory role of subtle vitamin B_{12} malabsorption. *Annals of International Medicine*, 1978; 88: 647.

Carter, J. P., Kattob, A., Abd-El-Hadi, K., Davis, J. T., El Cholmy, A., and Pathwardhan, V. N. Chromium III in hypoglycemia and impaired glucose utilization in Kwashiorkor. *American Journal of Clinical Nutrition*, 1968; 21: 195–202.

Chakravarthy, B. K., et al. Functional beta cell regeneration in the islets of pancreas in alloxan-induced diabetic rats by epicatechin. *Life Sciences*, 1982; 31240: 2693–97.

Chandalia, M., et al. Beneficial effects of high dietary fiber intake in patients with Type II diabetes mellitus. *New England Journal of Medicine*, 2000; 342(19): 1392–98.

Chaney, M. S., and Ross, M. L. *Nutrition*. Boston: Houghton Mifflin, 1971, p. 307.

Chen, P. *Soybeans for Health, Longevity, and Economy*. St. Catherines, Ontario: Provoker Press, 1970, p. 99.

Chromium metabolism in man and biochemical effects. In A. Prasad, ed., *Trace Elements in Human Health and Disease*. New York: Academic Press, vol. 2, ch. 29.

Clapp, A. Report on Medical Botany . . . A Synopsis, of systematic catalogue of the indigenous and naturalized, flowering and filicoid . . . medicinal plants of the United States. *Transactions of the American Medical Association*, Philadelphia, 1852, vol. V.

Clark, Linda. *Know Your Nutrition.* New Canaan, CT: Keats Publishing, 1973, p. 78.

Cleary, J. P. Vitamin B_3 in the treatment of diabetes mellitus. Case reports and review of the literature. *Journal of Nutritional Medicine,* 1990: 1: 217–25.

Coggershall, J. C., et al. Biotin status and plasma glucose in diabetics. *Annals of the New York Academy of Sciences,* 1985: 447: 389–92.

Colette, C., et al. Platelet function in Type I diabetes: Effects of supplementation with large doses of vitamin E. *American Journal of Clinical Nutrition,* 1988; 47: 256–61.

Collier, G. Effect of physical form of carbohydrate on the postprandial glucose, insulin and gastric inhibitory polypeptide responses in Type 2 diabetes. *American Journal of Clinical Nutrition,* 1982, 36: 10.

Connor, P. Nutritional vitamin B_{12} deficiency. *Medical Journal of Australia,* 1963; 2: 451.

Connor, W. The key role of nutritional factors in the prevention of coronary heart disease. *Preventive Medicine,* 1972; 1: 49.

Coustan, D. R. A randomized clinical trial of the insulin pump vs. intensive conventional therapy in diabetic pregnancies. *Journal of the American Medical Association,* 1978; 255: 631–36.

Culbreth, D. M. R. *A Manual of Materia Medica and Pharmacology.* Philadelphia, 1927.

Cullen, C. Intravascular aggregation and adhesiveness of the blood elements associated with alimentary lipemia and injections of large molecular substances. *Circulation,* 1954; 9: 335.

Cunnick, J., Takemoto, D., et al. Bitter melon (Momordica charantia). *Journal of Naturopathic Medicine,* 1993; 4: 16–21.

Dahl, L. Salt intake and salt need. *New England Journal of Medicine,* 1958; 258: 1152, 1205.

Dahlquist, G. G., et al. Dietary factors and the risk of developing insulin-dependent diabetes in childhood. *British Medical Journal,* 1990; 300: 1302–6.

Davidson, P. Insulin resistance in hyperglyceridemia. *Metabolism,* 1965; 14: 1059.

Davidson, S. The use of vitamin B_{12} in the treatment of diabetic neuropathy. *Journal of the Florida Medical Association,* 1954; 15: 717–20.

DCCT and Research Group. The effect of intensive treatment of diabetes on the development and progression of long-term complications in insulin-dependent diabetes mellitus. *New England Journal of Medicine,* 1993; 329: 977–86.

DECODE study group. Glucose tolerance and mortality: comparison of WHO and American Diabetes Association diagnostic criteria. *Lancet,* 1999; 354: 617–21.

Ditzel, J. Oxygen transport impairment in diabetes. *Diabetes,* 1976; 25: 832–38.

Douillet, C., et al. A selenium supplement associated or not with vitamin E delays early renal lesions in experimental diabetes in rats. *Proceedings of the Society for Experimental Biology and Medicine,* 1996; 211: 323–31.

Drause, M. V., and Hunscher, M. A. *Food, Nutrition, and Diet Therapy,* 5th ed. Philadelphia: W. B. Saunders Co., 1972, p. 141.

Duffield, R. Treatment of hyperlipidemia retards progression of symptomatic femerol atherosclerosis. *Lancet,* 1983; 2: 639.

Durlach, J., and Collery, P. Magnesium and potassium in diabetes and carbohydrate metabolism. Review of the present status and recent results. *Magnesium,* 1984; 3: 315–23.

Eaton, S. B., et al. Paleolithic nutrition, a consideration of its nature and current implications. *New England Journal of Medicine,* 1985; 312(5): 283–89.

Ebon, M. *The Truth about Vitamin E.* New York: Bantam, 1972, p. 7.

Echte, W. Die Einwirkung von Weissdom-extrakten auf die dynamic des menschlichen herzens. (The effect of Hawthorn extracts on the dynamics of the human heart). *Aerztliche Forshung,* 1960; 1: 560–66.

Editorial. Coronary artery bypass surgery—Indications and limitations. *Lancet,* 1980; 2: 511.

Editorial. Keep taking your bran. *Lancet,* 1979; 1: 1175.

Elam, M. B., et al. Effect of niacin on lipid and lipoprotein levels and glycemic control in patients with diabetes mellitus and peripheral arterial disease: The ADMIT study: A randomized trial. Arterial Disease Multiple Intervention Trial. *Journal of the American Medical Association,* 2000; 284(10): 1263–70.

Elamin, A., and Tuvemo, T. Magnesium and insulin-dependent diabetes mellitus. *Diabetes Research and Clinical Practice*, 1990; 10: 203–9.

Ellenberg, M. Diabetes: current status of the revolving disease. *New York State Journal of Medicine*, 1977; 77: 62–67.

Elliott, R. B., et al. A population-based strategy to prevent insulin-dependent diabetes using nicotinamide. *Journal of Pediatric Endocrinology and Metabolism*, 1996; 9: 501–9.

———. Prevention of diabetes in normal school children. *Diabetes Research and Clinical Practice*, 1991; 14: S85.

Ellis, F. Angina and vegan diet. *American Heart Journal*, 1977; 93: 803.

Ellis, J. M., et al. A deficiency of vitamin B_6 is a plausible molecular basis of the retinopathy of patients with diabetes mellitus. *Biochemical and Biophysical Research Communications*, 1991; 179: 615–19.

Elson, D. F., and Meredith, M. Therapy for Type II diabetes mellitus. *Wisconsin Medical Journal*, 1998; 97: 49–54.

Eriksson, J. G. Exercise and the treatment of Type II diabetes mellitus: An update. *Sports Medicine*, 1999; 27(6): 381–91.

Evans, G. W., Roginski, E. E., and Mertz, W. 1973. Interaction of the glucose tolerance factor, with insulin. *Biochemistry and Bile Physics Research Community*, 1973; 50: 718–22.

Everwib, G. J., and Schrader, R. E. Abnormal glucose tolerance in magnesium space deficient guinea pigs. *Journal of Nutrition*, 1968; 94: 89–94.

Farnsworth, N. R., and Segelman, A. B. Hypoglycemic plants. *Till and Tile*, 1971; 52–55.

Farquhar, J. Glucose, insulin and triglyceride responses on high- and low-carbohydrate diets in man. *Journal of Clinical Investigation*, 1966; 45: 1648.

Faure, P., et al. Zinc and insulin sensitivity. *Biological Trace Element Research*, 1992; 32: 305–10.

Ford, E. S., et al. Diabetes mellitus and serum carotenoids: Findings from the third National Health and Nutrition Examination Survey. *American Journal of Epidemiology*, 1999; 149: 168–76.

Fox, M. R. S. The status of zinc in human nutrition. *World Review of Nutrition Diet*, 1970; 12: 208–26.

Freestone, S. Effect of coffee and cigarette smoking in blood pressure of untreated and diuretic-treated hypertensive patients. *American Journal of Medicine,* 1982; 73: 348.

Friday, K. E., et al. Omega-3 fatty acid supplementation has discordant effects on plasma glucose and lipoproteins in Type II diabetes. *Diabetes,* 1987; 36(Suppl. 1): 12A.

Friedman, M. Effect of unsaturated fats upon lipemia and conjunctival circulation. *Journal of the American Medical Association,* 1965; 193: 110.

———. Serum lipids and conjunctival circulation after fat ingestion in men exhibiting Type-A behavior pattern. *Circulation,* 1964; 29: 874.

Fuller, C. J., et al. RRR-alpha-tocopheryl acetate supplementation at pharmacologic doses decreases low-density-lipoprotein oxidative susceptibility but not protein glycation in patients with diabetes mellitus. *American Journal of Clinical Nutrition,* 1996; 63: 753–59.

Funayama, S., and Hikino, H. Hypertensive principle of laminaria and allied seaweeds. *Planta Medica,* 1991; pp. 29–33.

Gabbay, K. H. The sorbitol pathway and the complications of diabetes. *New England Journal of Medicine,* 1973; 288: 831–36.

Garg, A., and Grundy, S. M. Nicotinic acid therapy for dyslipidemia in non-insulin-dependent diabetes mellitus. *Journal of the American Medical Association,* 1990; 264: 723–26.

Gear, J. Symptomless diverticular diseases and intake of dietary fiber. *Lancet,* 1979; 1: 511.

Genta, V. Vitamin A deficiency enhances binding of benzo(a)pyrene to tracheal epithelial DNA. *Nature,* 1974; 247: 48.

Gerstien, H. C. Cow's milk exposure and Type I diabetes mellitus. *Diabetes Care,* 1994; 17: 13–19.

Gilliland, F. D., et al. Temporal trends in diabetes mortality among American Indians and Hispanics in New Mexico: Birth cohort and period effects. *American Journal of Epidemiology,* 1997; 145: 422–31.

Gleeson, M. Complications of dietary deficiency of vitamin B_{12} in young Caucasians. *Postgraduate Medical Journal,* 1974; 50: 462.

Glinsmann, W. H., and Mertz. Effect of trivalent chromium on glucose tolerance metabolism. *Metabolism,* 1966; 15: 510–20.

Goh, Y. K., et al. Effect of omega-3 fatty acid on plasma lipids, cholesterol and lipoprotein fatty acid content in NIDDM patients. *Diabetologia,* 1997; 40: 45–52.

Goldfine, A. B., et al. Clinical trials of vanadium compounds in human diabetes mellitus. *Canadian Journal of Physiology and Pharmacology,* 1994; 72(Suppl. 3): 11.

Goldstein, D. E. How much do you know about glycated hemoglobin testing? *Clinical Diabetes,* July/August 1995, pp. 60–64.

Goodyear, L. J., and Kahn, B. B. Exercise, glucose transport, and insulin sensitivity. *Annual Review of Medicine,* 1998; 49: 235–61.

Greenbaum, C. J., et al. Nicotinamide's effect on glucose metabolism in subjects at risk for IDDM. *Diabetes,* 1996; 45: 1631–34.

Greig, H. Inhibition of fibrinolysis by alimentary lipemia. *Lancet,* 1956; 2: 16.

Gurson, C. T., and Saner, G. Effect of chromium on glucose utilization in marasmic protein-calorie malnutrition. *American Journal of Clinical Nutrition,* 1971; 24: 13.

Guthrie, B. E. Chromium, manganese, copper, sing, and cadmium content of New Zealand foods. *New Zealand Medical Journal,* 1975; 82: 418–24.

Guthrie, H. A. *Introductory Nutrition,* 2nd ed. St. Louis: C. V. Mosby Co., 1971, p. 262.

Halpern, R., and Smith, R. A. Molecular Biology Institute, as reported in Clark, *Know Your Nutrition,* p. 84.

Halsted, J. A., Smith, J. C., Jr., and Irwin, M. I. A prospectus of research on zinc requirements of man. *Journal of Nutrition,* 1975; 104: 347–78.

Hamberg, M. Thromboxanes: A new group of biologically active compounds derived from prostaglandin endoperoxides. *Procedures of the National Academy of Science,* 1975; 72: 2994.

Hambidge, K. M., Hambidge, C., Jacobs, M., and Baum, J. D. Low levels of zinc in hair, anorexia, poor growth, and high hypogenusia in children. *Pediatric Research,* 1972; 6: 868–74.

Hammeri, H., Kranzi, C., Pichler, O., and Studiar, M. Klinisch experimentelle stoffwechseluntersuchungen mit einem crataegus extract. (Clinical and experimental investigations on metabolism with an extract of Crataegus). *Aerzliche Forschung,* 1967, pp. 261–70.

Hankin, J. H., Margen, S., and Goldsmith, N. F. Contribution of acidic water to calcium and magnesium intakes of adults. *Journal of the American Diabetic Association,* 1970; 56: 212–24.

Harrell, R. F. Effect of added thiamine on learning. As reported in Rodale and Staff, *The Health Seeker,* pp. 18–19.

Herbert, V. The five possible causes of all nutrient deficiency, illustrated by deficiencies of vitamin B_{12} and folic acid. *American Journal of Clinical Nutrition,* 1973; 26: 77.

Heyssel, R. Vitamin B_{12} turnover in man. *American Journal of Clinical Nutrition,* 1966; 18: 176.

Higginbottom, M. A syndrome of methylmalonic aciduria, homocystinuria, megaloblastic anemia, and neurological abnormalities in a vitamin B_{12} breast-fed infant of a strict vegetarian. *New England Journal of Medicine,* 1978; 299: 317.

High polysaccharide diet studies in patients with diabetes and vascular disease. *Cereal Foods World;* 22: 12–15.

Hines, J. Megaloblastic anemia in an adult vegan. *American Journal of Clinical Nutrition,* 1966; 19: 260.

Hinsworth, H. Physiological activation of insulin. *Clinical Science,* 1933; 1: 1.

Hjermann, I. Effect of diet and smoking intravention on the incidence of coronary heart disease, report from the Oslo Study Group of a randomized trial in healthy men. *Lancet,* 1981; 2: 1303.

Hockerts, T., and Muelke, G. The coronary effect of aqueous extracts of Crataegus. *Arzneimittel-Forschungen,* 1955, pp. 755–57.

HogenKamp, H. Editorial: The interaction between vitamin B_{12} and vitamin C. *American Journal of Clinical Nutrition,* 1980; 33: 1.

Holman, R. Prevention of deterioration of renal and sensory-nerve function by more intensive management of insulin-dependent diabetic patients. *Lancet,* 1983; 1: 204.

Hoover, J. D., and Dunne, L. *Nutrition Almanac,* 2nd ed. New York: McGraw-Hill, 1984, p. 20.

Hopkins, L. L., Jr., Ransome-Kuti, O., and Majaf, A. S. Improvement of impaired carbohydrate metabolism by chromium III in malnourished infants. *American Journal of Clinical Nutrition,* 1968; 21: 203–11.

Hornstra, G. Influence of dietary fat on platelet function in men. *Lancet,* 1973; 1: 1155.

Horwitt, M. K., et al. Investigations of human requirements of B-complex vitamins. *National Research Council Bulletin,* 1948, p. 116.

Hounsom, L., et al. A lipoic acid-gamma linolenic acid conjugate is effective against multiple indices of experimental diabetic neuropathy. *Diabetologia,* 1998; 41: 839–43.

Hsia, S. L., Fishman, L/M., Briese, F. W.; Christakes, G., Burr, J., and Bricker, L. A. Decreases in serum cholesterol binding reserve in diabetes myelitis. *Diabetes Care,* 1978; 89–93.

Hsu, J. M., Davis, R. L., and Neithamer, R. W. Chromium and diabetes in the aged. In *The Biomedical Role of Trace Elements in Aging* (pp. 117–26). St. Petersburg, Fla.: Eckerd College Gerontology Center, 1976.

Hu, F. B., et al. Walking compared with vigorous physical activity and risk of Type 2 diabetes in women: A prospective study. *Journal of the American Medical Association,* 1999; 282(15): 1433–39.

Ippoliti, A. The effect of various forms of milk on gastric-acid secretions, studies in patients with duodenal ulcer and normal subjects. *Annals of International Medicine,* 1976; 84: 286.

Isaev, I., and Bojadzieva, M. Obtaining galenic and neogalenic preparations and experiments for the isolation of an active substance from leonurus cardiaca. *Nauchnye Trydy Nisshiia Meditsinski Institut* (Sofia), 1960, pp. 145–52.

Jacobson, M. F., et al. Liquid candy: How soft drinks are harming Americans' health. Center for Science in the Public Interest; http://www.cspinet.org/sodapop/liquid_candy.htm.

Jain, S. K., et al. Effect of modest vitamin E supplementation on blood glycated hemoglobin and triglyceride levels and red cell indices in Type I diabetic patients. *Journal of the American College of Nutrition,* 1996; 15: 458–61.

Jamal, G. A., Carmichael, H. The effect of gamma-linolenic acid on human diabetic peripheral neuropathy: a double-blind, placebo-controlled trial. *Diabetes Medicine,* 1990; 7: 319–323.

Jenkins, D. The diabetic diet, dietary carbohydrate and differences in digestibility. *Diabetologia,* 1982; 23: 477.

Jenkins, D. J. A., Leeds, A. R., Gassull, M. A., Cochet, B., and Alberti, K. G. M. M. Decrease in postprandial insulin and glucose concentrations by guar and pectin. *Annals of Internal Medicine,* 1977; 86: 20–23.

Jenkins, D. J. A., Leeds, A. R., Gassull, M. A., Wolever, T. D. R., Goff, D. V., Alberti, K. G. M. M., and Hockaday, T. D. R. Unabsorbable carbohydrates and diabetes: Decreased postprandial hyperglycemia. *Lancet,* 1976; 2: 172–74.

Jensen, T., et al. Partial normalization by dietary cod-liver oil of increased microvascular albumin leakage in patients with insulin-dependent diabetes and albuminuria. *New England Journal of Medicine,* 1989; 321: 1572–77.

Josselyn, J. New England's rarities discovered in birds, beasts, fishes, serpents, and plates of that country. *Archaeologica Americans,* Transaction and Collections of the American Antiquarian Society, Boston, 1860; vol. IV, pp. 105–238.

Journal of the American Medical Association, 1958; 167: 1806, as reported in Rodale, *The Encyclopedia for Healthful Living,* p. 980.

Kameda, J. Medical studies on sea weeds. I. *Fukushima Igaku Zassi,* pp. 289–309.

———. Medical studies on seaweeds. II. Influence of tangle administration on experimental rabbit atherosclerosis produced by cholesterol feeding. *Fukushima Igaku Zasshi,* 1960; p. 251.

Kanabrocki, E. L., Case, L. F., Graham, L., Fields, T., Miller, E. B., Oester, Y. T., and Kaplan, E. Non-dialyzable manganese and copper levels in serum of patients with various diseases. *Journal of Nuclear Medicine,* 1967; 8: 166–72.

Kandziora, J. Crataegutt-wirkung bei koronaren durchblutungsstoerungen. *Muenghener Medizinischer Wochenschrift,* 1960, pp. 295–98.

Kanner, J., Harel, S., and Mendel, H. Content and stability of alpha-tocopherols in fresh and dehydrated pepper fruits (Capsicum annum L). *Journal of Agriculture and Food Chemistry,* 1979.

Karjalainen, J., et al. A bovine albumin peptide as a possible trigger of insulin-dependent diabetes. *New England Journal of Medicine,* 1992; 327: 302–7.

Keen, H., et al. Treatment of diabetic neuropathy with gamma-linoleic acid. The Gamma-Linoleic Acid Multi-center Trial Group. *Diabetes Care,* 1993; 16: 8–15.

Kempner, W. The effect of rice diet on diabetes mellitus associated with vascular disease. *Postgraduate Medicine,* 1958; 24: 359.

Keys, A. Serum cholesterol response to changes in dietary lipids. *American Journal of Clinical Nutrition,* 1966; 19: 175 (1966).

———. Effects of different fats on blood coagulation. *Circulation,* 1957; 15: 274.

Khan, M. A., et al. Vitamin B_{12} deficiency and diabetic neuropathy. *Lancet,* 1969; 2: 769–70.

Kikkila, E. Prevention of progression of coronary atherosclerosis by treatment of hyperlipidemia: A seven-year prospective angiographic study. *British Medical Journal,* 1984; 289: 220.

Kirschmann, J. D., and Dunn, L. *Nutrition Almanac,* 2nd ed. New York: McGraw-Hill, 1984, pp. 13–15, 54, 241–81.

Kirwan, J. P., et al. Regular exercise enhances insulin activation of IRS-1-associated P13-kinase in human skeletal muscle. *Journal of Applied Physiology,* 2000; 88(2):797–803.

Klachko, D. M., et al. Blood glucose levels during walking in normal and diabetic subjects. *Diabetes,* 1972; 21: 89–100.

Klemes, I. S. Industrial medicine and surgery (June 1957), as reported in Rodale, *Encyclopedia for Healthful Living,* pp. 108–10.

Kohler, F. P., and Uhle, C. A. W. *Journal of Urology,* November 1966, as reported in Rodale, *Complete Book of Minerals for Health,* p. 78.

Kolata, G. Dietary dogma disproved. *Science,* 1983; 220: 487.

———. Consensus on bypass surgery. *Science,* 1981; 211: 42.

Kosenko, L. G. *Klinical Medizine,* 1964; 42: 113.

Kosuge, T., Nukaya, H., Yamamoto, T., and Tsuji, K. Isolation and identification of cardiac principles from laminaria. *Yakugaku Zasshi,* 1983, pp. 683–85.

Koutsikos, D., et al. Biotin for diabetic peripheral neuropathy. *Biomedicine and Pharmacotherapy,* 1990; 44: 511–14.

Kovach, A. G. B., Foldi, M., and Fedina, L. Die Wirkung eines extraktes aus Crataegus oxuacantha aufg die durchstromung der coronarien von hunden. (The effect of extracts from C. oxyacantha on the coronary circulation of dogs.) *Arzneimittel Forschung,* 1959.

Koya, D., et al. Prevention of glomerular dysfunction in diabetic rats by treatment with d-alpha-tocopherol. *Journal of the American Society of Nephrology,* 1997; 8: 426–35.

Krhel, W. A. *American Journal of Clinical Nutrition,* 1962; 11: 77.

Kubota, S. The study of leonurus sibericus L II. Pharmacological study of the alkaloid "leonurin" isolated from leonurus sibericus L. *Folia Pharmacologica Japonica,* pp. 159–167.

Kunisake, M., et al. Prevention of diabetes-induced abnormal retinal blood flow by treatment with d-alpha-tocopherol. *Biofactors,* 1998; 7: 55–67.

Kuo, P. The effect of lipemia upon coronary and peripheral arterial circulation in patients with essential hyperlipemia. *American Journal of Medicine,* 1959; 26: 68.

————. Lipemia in patients with coronary heart disease, treatment with low-fat diet. *Journal of the American Dietitians Association,* 1957; 33: 22.

————. Angina pectoris induced by fat ingestion in patients with coronary artery disease. *Journal of the American Dietitians Association,* 1955; 158: 1008.

Lampeter, E. F., et al. The Deutsche nicotinamide intervention study: An attempt to prevent Type I diabetes. DENIS Group. *Diabetes,* 1998; 47; 980–84.

Lampman, R. Comparative effectiveness of physical training and diet in normalizing serum lipids in men with Type IV hyperlipoproteinemia. *Circulation,* 1977; 55: 652.

Lappe, F. *Diet for a Small Planet,* New York: Galantine Books, 1971, p. 88.

Larharl, K. D. *Journal of the Indian Medical Association* (March 1954), as reported in Rodale, ed., *Prevention* (November 1968).

La Riforma Medical, 1955; 69: 853–56, as reported in Rodale, *Encyclopedia for Healthful Living,* p. 978.

Leatherdale, B. A., et al. Improvement of glucose tolerance due to

Momordica charantia (Karela). *British Medical Journal (Clinical Research Ed)*, 1981; 282: 1823–24.

Ledbetter, R. Severe megaloblastic anemia due to nutritional B_{12} deficiency. *Acta Haemat*, 1969; 42: 247.

Leek, S. *Herbs, Medicine and Mysticism.* Chicago: Henry Regnery Co., 1975.

Leslie, R. D. G., et al. Early environmental events as a cause of IDDM. *Diabetes*, 1994; 43: 843–50.

Leung, A. Y. *Encyclopedia of Common Natural Ingredients.* New York: Wiley-Interscience, 1980, pp. 257–59.

Levin, E. R., et al. The influence of pyridoxine in diabetic peripheral neuropathy. *Diabetes Care*, 1981; 4: 606–9.

Levine, R. A., Streeten, D. H. P., and Doisy, R. J. 1968. Effects of oral chromium supplementation on the glucose tolerance of elderly human subjects. *Metabolism*, 1968; 17: 114–25.

Levy-Marchal, C., et al. Antibodies against bovine albuim and other diabetic markers in French children. *Diabetes Care*, 1995; 18: 1089–94.

Lewis, W. H., and Elvin-Lewis, M. P. F. *Medical Botany.* New York: John Wiley & Sons, 1977.

Li, Shih-chen. *Chinese Medicinal Herbs*, translated by F. Porter Smith and G. A. Stuart. San Francisco: Georgetown Press, 1973.

Linday, L. A. Trivalent chromium and the diabetes prevention program. *Med Hypotheses*, 1997; 49: 47–49.

Linnell, J. Effects of smoking on metabolism and excretion of vitamin B_{12}. *British Medical Journal*, 1968; 2: 215.

List, P. H., and Hoerhammer, L. *Hagers Handbuch der Pharmazeutischen Praxis*, vols. 2–5. Berlin: Springer-Verlag.

Long term effects of high carbohydrate, high fiber diets on glucose and lipid metabolism: A preliminary report on patients with diabetes. *Diabetes Care*, 1: 77082.

Lostroh, A. J., and Krahl, M. E. Magnesium, a second messenger for insulin: Ion translocation coupled to transport activity. *Advances in Enzyme Regulation*, 1974; 12: 73–81.

Lubin, B., Machlin, L. Biological aspects of vitamin E. *Annals of the New York Academy of Sciences*, 1982, p. 393.

Lust, J. *The Herb Book.* Simi Valley, CA: Benedict Lust, 1974.

Madsen, J. L., *Journal of Animal Science,* as reported in Rodale, ed., *Prevention* (January 1971).

Maebashi, M., et al. Therapeutic evaluation of the effect of biotin on hyperglycemia in patients with non-insulin-dependent diabetes mellitus. *Journal of Clinical Biochemical Nutrition,* 1993; 14: 211–18.

Mann, D. Appropriate cardiovascular therapy: Clinical and experimental study of the action of an injectable preparation of crataegus. *Zeitschrift fuer die Gesamte Innere Medizin und Ihre Grenzgbiete,* 1963, pp. 145–51.

Martindale. *The Extra Pharmacopoeia,* London: The Pharmaceutical Press, 1977.

Mateo, M. C., et al. Serum zinc, copper and insulin in diabetes mellitus. *Biomedicine,* 1978; 29: 56–58.

Mather, H. M. Hypomagnesaemia in diabetes. *Acta Clinica Chemica,* 1979; 95: 235–42.

Mathew, P. T., and Augusti, K. T. Hypoglycaemic effects of onion, Allium cepa Linn. on diabetes mellitus—A preliminary report. *Indian Journal of Physiology and Pharmacology,* 1975; 19: 213–17.

Mayer-Davis, E. J. Intensity and amount of physical activity in relation to insulin sensitivity. *Journal of the American Medical Association,* 1998; 279(9): 669–74.

McCance and Widdowson. *The Composition of Foods.* Medical Research Council Special Report series no. 297, Her Majesty's Stationery Office, London, England.

Mcintosh, H. The first decade of aortocoronary bypass grafting, 1967–1977, a review. *Circulation,* 1978; 57: 405.

McNair, P., et al. Hypomagnesium, a risk factor in diabetic retinopathy. *Diabetes,* 1978: 27: 1075–77.

Mertz, W. Biological role of chromium. *Federation Proceedings,* 1967; 26: 186–93.

Mettlin, C. Dietary risk factors in human bladder cancer. *American Journal of Epidemiology,* 1979; 110: 255.

Millspaugh, C. F. *American Medicinal Plants.* New York: Dover, 1974.

Misra, H. Subacute combined degeneration of the spinal cord in a vegan. *Postgraduate Medical Journal,* 1971; 47: 624.

Montori, V. M., et al. Fish oil supplementation in Type II diabetes: A quantitative systemic review. *Diabetes Care,* 2000; 23: 1407–15.

Mooradian, A. G., et al. Selected vitamins and minerals in diabetes. *Diabetes Care,* May 1994; 341(4): 464–479.

Moore, F. D., et al. *Metabolism,* 1955; 4: 379.

Morales, Betty Lee, ed., *Cancer Control Journal,* 1974; 2: 3: 13.

Morgan, A. F., et al. *Journal of Biological Chemistry,* 1952; 195: 583.

Morgan, J. M. 1972. Hepatic chromium content in diabetic subjects. *Metabolism,* 1972; 21: 313–16.

Morrison, Cr. L. M., and Gonzalez, W. F. *Proceedings of the Society of Biology and Medicine,* 1950; 73: 37–38, as reported in Rodale, *Encyclopedia for Healthful Living,* pp. 457–58.

Murphy, M. Vitamin B_{12} deficiency due to a low-cholesterol diet in vegetarian. *Annals of International Medicine,* 1981; 94: 57.

Mustard, J. Effect of different fats on blood coagulation, platelet economy, and blood lipids. *British Medical Journal,* 1962; 2: 1651.

Muth, H. W. Studies on the vasoactive effects of Cratemon preparations. *Therapie Der Gegenwart,* 1976, pp. 242–55.

Nickander, K. K., et al. Alpha-lipoic acid: antioxidant potency against lipid peroxidation of neural tissues in vitro and implications for diabetic neuropathy. *Free Radical Biology and Medicine,* 1996; 21: 631–39.

O'Brian, J. Fat ingestion, blood coagulation, and atherosclerosis. *American Journal of Medical Science,* 1957; 234: 373.

O'Brien, J. Acute platelet changes after large meals of saturated and unsaturated fats. *Lancet,* 1976; 1: 878.

O'Dea, K. Physical factors influencing postprandial glucose and insulin responses to starch. *American Journal of Clinical Nutrition,* 1971; 33: 521.

O'Dell, B. L., Morris, E. R., and Reagan, W. O. Magnesium requirements of guinea pigs and rats. Effects of calcium and phosphorus and symptoms of magnesium deficiency. *Journal of Nutrition,* 1960; 70: 103–11.

Olefsky, J. Reappraisal of the role of insulin in hypertriglyceridemia. *American Journal of Medicine,* 1974; 57: 551.

Oliva, P. Pathophysiology of acute myocardial infarction, 1981. *Annals of International Medicine,* 1981; 94: 236.

Omish, D. Effects of stress management training and dietary change in treating ischemic heart disease. *Journal of the American Medical Association,* 1983; 249: 54.

Onuma, T., et al. Effect of vitamin E on plasma lipoprotein abnormalities in diabetic rats. *Diabetes, Nutrition and Metabolism,* 1993; 6: 135–38.

Ornish, D., et al. Can lifestyle changes reverse coronary heart disease? The lifestyle heart trial. *Lancet,* 1990; 336: 129–33.

Ozawa, H., Gomi, Y., and Otsudi, I. Pharmacological studies on laminine monocitrate. *Yakugaku Zasshi,* 1967, pp. 935–39.

Pai, L. H., and Prasad, A. Cellular zinc in patients with diabetes mellitus. *Nutrition Research,* 1988; 8: 889–98.

Painter, N. The high-fiber diet in the treatment of diverticular disease of the colon. *Postgraduate Medical Journal,* 1974; 50: 629.

Paolisso, G., et al. Improved insulin response and action by chronic magnesium administration in aged NIDDM subjects. *Diabetes Care,* 1989; 12: 265–69.

Pedersen, M. *Nutritional Herbology.* Bountiful, UT: Petersen Publishing, 1988, p. 149.

Pedersen, O. Increased insulin receptors after exercise in patients with insulin-dependent diabetes mellitus. *New England Journal of Medicine,* 1980; 302: 886–92.

Peer, L. A. 22nd Annual Meeting of International College of Surgeons, as reported in Rodale, *The Health Seeker,* p. 194.

Perex, G. O., et al. Potassium homeostasis in chronic diabetes mellitus. *Archives of Internal Medicine,* 1977; 137: 1018–22.

Peto, R. Can dietary beta-carotene materially reduce human cancer rates? *Nature,* 1981; 290: 201.

Podrid, P. Prognosis of medically treated patients with coronary-artery disease with profound ST-segment depression during exercise testing. *New England Journal of Medicine,* 1981; 305: 1111.

Pollack, H., et al. *Therapeutic Nutrition.* Publication #234, National Research Council, 1952.

Polyadov, N. G. A study of the biological activity of infusions of valerian and motherwort and their mixtures. *Information of the First All-Russian Session of Pharamacists,* Moscow, 1964, pp. 319–24.

Pozzilli, P., et al. Meta-analysis of nicotinamide treatment in patients with recent-onset IDDM. The Nicotinamide Trialists. *Diabetes Care*, 1996; 19: 1357–63.

————. Double blind trial of nicotinamide treatment in recent-onset IDDM (the IMDIAB III study). *Diabetologia*, 1995; 38: 848–52.

Prakash, A. O., et al. Effects of feeding Gymnema sylvestre leaves on blood glucose in beryllium nitrate treated rats. *Journal of Ethnopharmacology*, 1986; 18: 143–46.

Prasad, G. Studies on etiopathogenesis of hemorrhoids. *American Journal of Proctology*, June 1976, p. 33.

Pritkin, N. *Research Projects*. Santa Monica, CA: Pritkin Research Foundation, 1981.

Public Citizen's Health Research Group. Risk of serious low blood sugar with antidiabetic drugs. *Worst Pills Best Pills News*, Dec. 1996; 2(12): 46.

————. Acarbose (Precose) for diabetcs no substitute for diet and exercise. *Worst Pills Best Pills*, April 1996; 2(6): 14.

Ralli, I. P. *Nutritional Symposium Series*, 1952; 5: 78.

Ramanadham, S., et al. Oral vanabyl sulfate in the treatment of diabetes mellitus in rats. *American Journal of Physiology*, 1989; 257: 904–11.

Ravina A., et al. Clinical use of the trace element chromium (III) in the treatment of diabetes mellitus. *Journal of Trace Elements in Medicine and Biology*, 1985; 8: 183–90.

Ravina, A., and Slezak, L. Chromium in the treatment of clinical diabetes mellitus (in Hebrew). *Harefuah*, 1993; 125(5-6): 142–45.

Raz, I., et al. The influence of zinc supplementation on glucose homeostasis in NIDDM. *Diabetes Res*, 1980; 11: 73–79.

Reaven, G. M. *Syndrome X: Overcoming the Silent Killer That Can Give You a Heart Attack*. New York: Simon & Schuster, 2000.

————. Role of insulin resistance in human disease. *Diabetes*, 1988; 37: 1595–1607.

————. Effects of differences on amount and kind of dietary carbohydrate on plasma glucose and insulin responses in man. *American Journal of Clinical Nutrition*, 1979; 32: 2568.

Reuters Health Information, Inc. High sugar intake ups heart risk. June 22, 1998; http://www.reutershealth.com.

Rewerksi, W., and Lewark, S. Hypotonic and sedative polyphenol and procyanidin extracts from hawthorn. *Ger. Offen,* 1970; 2: 145–211.

———. Pharmacological properties of flaven polymers isolated from hawthorn (crataegus oxyacantha). *Arzneimittel-Forschungen,* 1967, pp. 490–91.

Rewerksi, W., Tadeusz, P., Rylski, M., and Lewark, S. Pharmacological properties of oligomeric procyanidin crataegus oxyacantha (hawthorn). *Arzneimittel-Forschungen,* 1971, pp. 886–88.

Ribes, G., et al. Antidiabetic effects of subfractions from fenugreek seeds in diabetic dogs. *Proceedings of the Society for Experimental Biology and Medicine,* 1986; 182: 159–66.

Rimm, E. B. Vitamin E consumption and the risk of coronary disease in men. *New England Journal of Medicine,* 1993; 328: 1450–55.

Rodale, J. I. *The Encyclopedia for Healthful Living.* Emmaus, PA: Rodale Books, 1970, p. 117.

———. *The Health Seeker.* Emmaus, PA: Rodale Books, 1962, p. 869.

Rumessen, J. J., et al. Fructans of Jerusalem artichokes: Intestinal transport, absorption, fermentation, and influence on blood glucose, insulin, and C-peptide responses in healthy subjects. *American Journal of Clinical Nutrition,* 1990; 52: 675–84.

Sadritdinov, F. Comparative study of the anti-inflammatory properties of alkaloids from gentiana plants. *Farmakologia Alkaloidov Serdechnykh Glikozidov,* 1971, pp. 146–48.

Saudek, C. D., and Brach, E. L. Cholesterol metabolism in diabetes. The effect of diabetic control on sterol balance. *Diabetes,* 1987; 27: 1059–64.

Saudek, C. D., et al. *The Johns Hopkins Guide to Diabetes for Today and Tomorrow.* Baltimore: John Hopkins University Press, 1997, pp. 22–29.

Schauenburg, P., and Paris, F. *Guide to Medicinal Plants.* Guildford, UK: Keats Publishing, 1977.

Searl, P. B., Norton, T. R., and Lum, B. K. B. Study of a cardiotonic fraction from an extract of the seaweed, Undaria pinnatifida. *Proceedings of the Western Pharmacology Society,* 1981, pp. 63–65.

Seltzer, H. S. Diagnosis of diabetes. In S. S. Fajans and K. E. Sussmand, eds., *Diabetes Mellitus: Diagnosis and Treatment.* New York: McGraw-Hill, 1979, pp. 436–507.

Selye, H. *The Stress of Life.* New York: McGraw-Hill, 1956.

———. *Journal of Clinical Endocrinology,* 1946; 6: 117.

Shamberger, R.J. The insulin-like effects of vanadium. *Journal of Advanced Medicine,* 1996; 9: 121–31.

Shanmugasundarum, E. R., et al. Possible regeneration of the islets of Langerhans in streptozotocin-diabetic rats given Gymnema sylvestre leaf extracts. *Journal of Ethnopharmacology,* 1990; 30: 265–79.

———. Use of Gymnema sylvestre leaf extract in the control of blood glucose in insulin dependent diabetes mellitus. *Journal of Ethnopharmacology,* 1990; 30: 281–94.

Sharma, R. D., et al. Effect of fenugreek seeds on blood glucose and serum lipids in Type I diabetes. *European Journal of Clinical Nutrition,* 1990; 44: 301–6.

Shekelle, R. Dietary Vitamin A and risk of cancer in the Western Electric Study. *Lancet,* 1981; 2: 1185.

Shimizu, K. Suppression of glucose absorption by some fractions extracted from Gymnema sylvestre leaves. *Journal of Veterinary Medicine Science,* 1997; 59(4): 245–51.

Shoemaker, J. V. *A Practical Treatise on Materia Medica and Therapeutics.* Philadelphia, 1908, p. 910.

Shun, D. Nutritional megalobalistic anemia in vegan. *New York State Journal of Medicine,* 1972; 2: 2893.

Shute, W. E., and Taub, H. J. *Vitamin E for Ailing and Healthy Hearts.* New York: Pyramid House, 1969, pp. 75–77.

Silver, A. A., and Krantz, J. C. The effect of the ingestion of burdock root on normal and diabetic individuals. A preliminary report. *Annals of Internal Medicine,* 1931; 5: 274–84.

Singh, I. Low-fat diet and therapeutic doses of insulin in diabetes mellitus. *Lancet,* 1955; 1: 422.

Sjogren, A., et al. Magnesium, potassium and zinc deficiency in subjects with Type II diabetes mellitus. *Acta Medicica Scandinavica,* 1988; 224: 461–66.

Smith, A. Veganism: A clinical survey with observations of vitamin B_{12} metabolism. *British Medical Journal,* 1962; 1: 1655.

Sokoloff, Boris. *Cancer: New Approaches, New Hope.* New York: Devin-Adair.

Soman, V. Increased insulin sensitivity and insulin binding to monocytes after physical training. *New England Journal of Medicine,* 1979; 301: 1200.

Sporn, M. Prevention of chemical cardinogenesis by vitamin A and its synthetic analogs (retinoids). *Federal Proceedings,* 1976; 35: 1332.

Stamler, J. Lifestyles, major risk factors, proof and public policy. *Circulation,* 1978; 53: 3.

Stampfer, M. J., et al. Vitamin E consumption and the risk of coronary disease in women. *New England Journal of Medicine,* 1993; 328: 1444–48.

Stewart, J. Response of dietary vitamin B_{12} deficiency to physiological oral doses of cyanocobalamin. *Lancet,* 1970; 2: 542.

Straumfjord, J. V. Astoria, Oregon, as reported in Rodale, ed., *Prevention* (November 1968).

Strom, A. Mortality from circulatory diseases in Norway 1940–1945. *Lancet,* 1951; 1: 126.

Sweeney, S. Dietary factors that influence the dextrose tolerance test. *Archives of International Medicine,* 1927; 40: 818.

Trowell, H. Definition of dietary fiber and hypotheses that it is a protective factor in certain diseases. *American Journal of Clinical Nutrition,* 1976; 29: 417.

Turova, M. A. *Lekarstvennye Sredstava Lz Rastenyi (Medical-Herbal Preparations).* Moscow: Medicinskaya Leteratura, 1962.

Tyler, V. E., et al. *Pharmacognosy,* 7th ed. Philadelphia: Lea & Febiger, 1976.

Ullsperger, R. Vorlaufige mitteilung ueber den coronargefaesse erweiternden wirkkoerper aus weissdom. (Preliminary communication concerning a coronary vessel dilating principle from hawthorn). *Pharmazie,* 1951, pp. 141–44.

Vague, P., et al. Effect of nicotinamide treatment on the residual insulin secretion in Type I (insulin-dependent) diabetic patients. *Diabetologia*, 1989; 32: 316–21.

Van Eck, W. The effect of a low-fat diet on the serum lipids in diabetes and its significance in diabetic retinopathy. *American Journal of Medicine*, 1959; 27: 196.

Varma, S. D., et al. Refractive change in alloxan diabetic rabbits, controlled by flavonoids I. *Acta Opthalmologica*, 1980; 58: 748–59.

Vitamin B₆: The Doctors Report. New York: Harper and Row, 1973.

Wald, N. Low serum—Vitamin A and subsequent risk of cancer, preliminary results of a prospective study. *Lancet*, 1980; 2: 813.

Walker, A. Appendicitis, fiber intake, and bowel behavior in ethnic groups in South Africa. *Postgraduate Medical Journal*, 1973; 49: 243.

Walker, K. Z., et al. Effects of regular walking on cardiovascular risk factors and body composition in normaoglycemic women and women with Type II diabetes. *Diabetes Care*, 1999; 22(4): 555–61.

Wapnick, S., Wicks, A. C. B., Kanengoni, E., and Jones, J. J. Can diet be responsible for the initial lesion in diabetes? *Lancet*, 1972; 2: 300–301.

Weisburger, J. Inhibition of carcinogenesis: Vitamin C and the prevention of gastric cancer. *Preventive Medicine*, 1980; 9: 352.

———. Nutrition and cancer—On the mechanisms bearing on causes of cancer of the colon, breast, prostate, and stomach. *Bulletin from the New York Academy of Medicine*, 1980; 56: 673.

Werbach, M. R., Murray, M. T. *Botanical Influences on Illness: A Sourcebook of Clinical Research*. Tarzana, CA: Third Line Press, 1994, p. 28.

West, E. The electroencephalogram in veganism, vegetarianism, vitamin B₁₂ deficiency, and in controls. *Journal of Neurological and Neurosurgical Psychiatry*, 1966; 29: 391.

West, K. M., and Kalbfleisch, J. M. Influence of nutritional factor on prevalence of diabetes. *Diabetes*, 1971; 20: 99–108.

Westlake, C. Appendectomy and dietary fiber. *Journal of Human Nutrition*, 1980; 34: 267.

Whitaker, J. *Reversing Heart Disease*. New York: Warner Books, 1985. Cited in *The Good Fats: Prevention's Guide to the Cholesterol-Fighting Omega-3 Oils*. Emmaus, PA: Rodale Press, Inc., 1988.

Williams, A. Increased blood cell agglutination following ingestion of fat, a factor contributing to cardiac ischemia, coronary insufficiency, and anginal pain. *Angiology,* 1957; 8: 29.

Williams, D. E., et al. Frequent salad vegetable consumption is associated with a reduction in the risk of diabetes mellitus. *Journal of Clinical Epidemiology,* 1999; 52(4): 329–35.

Williams, R. J., *Nutrition Against Disease.* New York: Pitman Publishing, 1971, pp. 75–76, 126.

Winawer, S. Gastric and hematological abnormalities in a vegan with nutritional B_{12} deficiency. Effects of oral vitamin B_{12}. *Gastroenterology,* 1967; 53: 130.

Womersley, R. A., et al. *Journal of Clinical Investigation,* 1955; 34: 456.

Wood, P. The distribution of plasma lipoproteins in middle-aged male runners. *Metabolism,* 1976; 25: 1249.

Xia, Y. X. The inhibitory effect of motherwort extract on pulsating myocardial cells in vitro. *Journal of Traditional Chinese Medicine,* 1983; 185–88.

Yaniv, Z., et al. Plants used for the treatment of diabetes in Israel. *Journal of Ethnopharmacology,* 1987; 19(2): 145–51.

Zang, C., et al. Studies of actions of extract of motherwort. *Journal of Traditional Chinese Medicine,* 1982, p. 267.

Index

About the Authors

ROBERT O. YOUNG, PH.D., D.SC., is a nationally renowned microbiologist and nutritionist who speaks to audiences around the world on health and wellness. He holds a degree in microbiology and nutrition and has devoted his life to researching the causes of disease and helping people reclaim their health and well-being. Dr. Young is head of the InnerLight Biological Research and Health Education Foundation and has gained national recognition for his research into diabetes, cancer, leukemia, and AIDS. He is a member of the American Society of Microbiologists and the American Naturopathic Association and conducts classes in live blood analysis and the "New Biology."

SHELLEY REDFORD YOUNG, L.M.T., is a licensed massage therapist with a passionate interest in optimum nutrition. With Dr. Young she speaks to audiences around the world on the basic requirements of a healthful diet, sharing her delicious, alkalizing, vegetarian recipes (many examples given in this book).

Together, Robert and Shelley Young provide a dynamic dose of health and nutrition expertise, guaranteed to inform and en*light*en.